Hypnosis

Learn the Secret Techniques and the
Exact Hypnotic Scripts to Hypnotize,
Persuade and Control Anyone

Leonard Moore

TABLE OF CONTENTS

Free Bonus:
3 Insanely Effective Words To Hypnotize Anyone in a Conversation

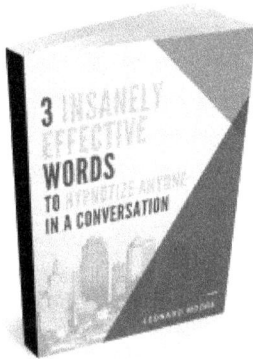

If you're trying to persuade and convince other people then words are the most important tool you absolutely have to master.

As humans we interact with words, we shape the way we think through words, we express ourselves through words. Words evoke feelings and have the ability to talk to the listener's subconscious.

In this free guide you'll discover 3 insanely effective words that you can easily use to start hypnotizing anyone in a conversation.

Go to **http://eepurl.com/cRTY5X** to download the free guide

Chapter One:
Power of Hypnosis

Hypnosis is and has been a prevalent part of pop culture ever since humans began to investigate the brain and its functions. The term comes from the Greek term "Hypnos", meaning "sleep". However, as hypnosis has changed and evolved along with its connotation, the literal translation has become a misnomer. A way of utilizing charisma, suggestion, and therapy to induce a uniquely human condition which we call trance, hypnosis has become an interesting and highly debated topic.

The idea of hypnosis first reached the public eye as we know it today in the late 1930s, although modern hypnosis itself was first introduced to the world of medicine in the late 18th century. As you can see, hypnosis has been relevant and present in the world for a very long time—it's not just a fad or a temporary bout of hysteria. No, hypnosis isn't nearly as magical as some may make it out to be. Hypnosis is a very scientific process which helps people to ease their pain, fight mental illness, and calm overall suffering in the lives of many. Hypnosis itself has evolved from a mysterious process to a stage show, a party trick—of course; it's also used more successfully in therapy now more than ever. This evolution of hypnosis and its allure in the media begs the question, why is it so interesting? What's so enrapturing about hypnosis?

The answer likely lies in why we are so fascinated with sleep and the afterlife. Although hypnosis has a little tether to what happens after we pass, it does represent the unknown. Because hypnosis is, although old, still a fairly new area of study new to its mystery in the world of medicine, we have yet to grasp it in its entirety. There are many scientists and researchers of hypnosis who posit many different theories every day having to do with hypnosis, hypnotic trance, induction, suggestion, and many other things. Because we understand fairly little about the process itself, we seek out more mystical explanations for it. Similar to the afterlife, we fill in areas where we have no answer with often fantastical ideas and possibilities.

Somewhere along the way, hypnosis developed from a mystical medicinal field to a sort of overdone party trick. This party trick, although often dramatized, can hold just as much power as therapeutic hypnosis. Although television and media have portrayed this sort of hypnosis as sinister or silly, recreational hypnosis has a fairly large following, and that recreational hypnosis fills in the gaps of actual experience or a medical degree, with placebo. The charisma and confidence of a hypnotist are what ultimately sells hypnosis as a therapeutic or recreational process, so those who are enraptured in the "performance" of the hypnotist pay less attention to any technical mistakes that might've been made. This is also why those who are more prone to daydreaming and those who focus easily are more susceptible to hypnosis and trance.

Hypnosis may also be considered a highly interesting topic to society now because we have a strange fascination with loss of control. Although hypnosis isn't technically any real loss of control in its entirety, we do cease to become totally autonomous and independent while in trance, so it may be that we're fascinated with that sensation. We're often plagued with stress in life, and ways to relieve that stress are marketed as heavily as water, soda, and candy. Hypnosis is a way to truly relieve stress in a very effective way, although temporarily—you can't be stressed over something if you've ceased to think thoughts the way we're used to. If we shut off the conscious mind and feed the subconscious only positive information, we remove most/ all sources of stress from the hypnotic subject for the duration of the session. Additionally, many hypnotists, both recreational and therapeutic, tend to add post-hypnotic suggestions which involve the subject still feeling relaxed focused, and happy, even after the session has ended. These suggestions can last any length of time depending on the suggestion and the subject. Some suggestions can last minutes, some can last weeks. Sometimes, those suggestions have to be removed by the very same hypnotist that placed it in the subject. However, if the subject is aware of it and very adamantly against the suggestion, most subjects can remove it themselves, or allow it to fade into the background of the subconscious mind.

That subconscious mind plays a massive role in the development of the relationship that inevitably builds and swells between a hypnotic subject and their hypnotist.

When the subconscious is bared that way, even if the exchange isn't at all meant to be romantic, the very experience itself is, by design, very intimate interaction between the two people. Hypnosis is often an experience that takes place more than once between the same pair of people, the same subject and hypnotist working together. Because these two people so often work with one another, the hypnotist and subject often grow much attached to one another. It can difficult, actually, to avoid building a connection with your subject as a hypnotist. Even as a beginner or novice hypnotist, all humans have at least a mild compulsion to take care of those around us. When we put a subject in trance and see the pure and raw trust that the subject has put into their hypnotist, we can't help but try our hardest to fulfill that trust, giving the subject a satisfying experience. That trust is a kind of latent function of hypnosis—the building of a relationship takes a back seat to the appeal of persuasion and control, but that relationship is never one that should be ignored by either party.

Hypnosis is, admittedly, not used as widely as the public fascination with any way to release stress would suggest. But, this may simply be because many people don't think hypnosis is real, to begin with. It also may be up to the fact that many therapists aren't licensed in hypnotherapy. Stress relief through hypnosis doesn't have to be sought out only through therapeutic practices, though. Recreational hypnosis brings most of the same components to the table —although in recreational hypnosis, the point is to focus on the subject's pleasure/fun, not helping a serious mental problem they may have, or trauma they may have repressed. It may be that when put in an environment where the hypnotist or partner is someone you trust more than a therapist you may not actually know, the subject has a much easier time relaxing and enjoying the experience.

Of course, there are some people who are simply too stressed out to go into trance properly. Those who suffer from chronic anxiety or stress to an extreme degree likely have much more trouble relaxing and focusing on one particular thing, so they would need a veteran or expert hypnotherapist to help them. There's no one who can't ever be hypnotized, but being in a state of panic for most of your life certainly doesn't help your case very much. If you're going into your first session of hypnosis, remember that what makes hypnosis actually work most of the time is the ability to relax and focus. These two things are the key to a successful and satisfying trance. Taking deep breaths and keeping your heart rate low are good first steps to prepare yourself to be hypnotized, especially since the first requests of a hypnotist are usually to being breathing deeply and calmly. It may help to count 3 seconds of an inhale and 5 seconds of an exhale, but different things work for different people.

Hypnosis remains today as a highly discussed topic, both in recreation and in therapy, and many people debate on whether or not hypnosis even exists. However, hypnosis gets its power from your mind and mine. The power of believing in hypnosis is the power that drives it to work in the first place. So, of course, if you don't believe in it, it ceases to exist. If you do believe in it, then hypnosis is as real as any other power of the world or of the mind. When you think about it in that sense, "mind over matter" proves itself to be true.

Chapter Two:
It Could Be Anyone of Us

There are many things that people often misunderstand about hypnosis. Hypnosis itself is a highly debated topic, as many people are still unconvinced that such a thing exists. Many believe that their mind isn't able to be hypnotized, or that only people with low intelligence can be put into a trance. Here are some popular misunderstandings about hypnosis, and the truth behind them;

- **Highly intelligent people can't be hypnotized**: Incorrect. In reality, those who are naturally more intelligent are also more susceptible to hypnosis and fall into trance more easily. On a connected note, more intelligent people are usually more able to meditate and more often find themselves daydreaming.

- **Hypnosis can make you do things against your will**: Actually, hypnosis is simply a state of heightened focus, so you can never be made to do things that you wouldn't otherwise do. To be technical, your actual desire can be changed under a trance, but only to an extent. The details of what you want or don't want can be changed, but your morals and can't. Your morals aren't things that can be suggested to another stance.

- **Being in trance is just like sleeping/gives the other person total control**: Being in a hypnotic trance allows for the hypnotist to plant suggestions into the mind of the subject, but the subject in trance doesn't lose all lucidity. Because hypnosis is a state of intense focus, the subject is in a mental state where they become passive listeners in their own bodies. Some hypnotic subjects aren't listening consciously to suggestions without being prompted, but some are. Whether or not your subject actively listens to suggestion can change the way you format your scripts and inductions. Additionally, if the subject is being asked or commanded to do something they wouldn't otherwise do in any situation; their subconscious can resist that suggestion. The ways that different subjects resist can vary, but most subjects will snap out of the trance, or at least "wake" part of the way up. Other subjects stay in trance, but simply ignore the suggestion entirely. If the subject ignores the suggestion, consider how much you had discussed boundaries with the subject before the session began.

- **Hypnosis turns people into vegetables/ zombies**: Because we often see hypnotic subjects become relatively unresponsive during hypnosis, we can often be drawn to the conclusion that a subject cannot respond and somehow loses sentience while hypnotized. However, most subjects do respond and recall most, if not all, information from when they were hypnotized. Often, the subject will remember most or all of the session in a foggy way, similarly to how we remember what is going on around us in the moments between being awake and falling asleep; we understand what's going on, but it becomes much more difficult to read between the lines and understand the context of things that happen. Although we focus more intensely than usual when we're hypnotized, we're also more relaxed than normal, so we tend to lose the details of things that happen while in trance.

- **You can be hypnotized anytime, anywhere**: This misconception lends itself to the stereotype that hypnosis is used to manipulate and control people, or for other malicious or sinister reasons. To be properly hypnotized, most subjects require a calm environment where they can relax and focus. Some subjects need more or less light than others, but no one can be put under trance if they're in a noisy and disruptive place. Also, it's much harder for someone to be hypnotized if they're in an unfamiliar environment or with an unfamiliar person, and most people go into trance more easily during the night hours.

- **Trance is the same for everyone:** Trance is usually much different for everyone who goes into it, and the experience is usually different every time. Someone who has an almost identical experience several times in trance may have a completely different experience the latest time. This can be due to changes at home, moving, new relationships, or stress, or nothing in particular. The human mind is fickle and can be made to change on a dime without much rhyme or reason. Different personalities can react differently to different suggestions, and different suggestions can be followed on one day and denied on the very next. Be careful every time you put a subject under a trance, and don't expect boundaries to hold fast for every session.

Hypnosis is a subject of a lot of public debate, ranging from the specifics to whether or not it even really exists. To some people, it doesn't exist and can never exist—you can't be hypnotized if you don't want to be. By design, hypnosis is an act that can only be carried out by two consenting individuals. When two people agree on boundaries and on what they want to happen, trance comes more easily to the subject, and control/guidance comes more easily to the hypnotist. And, of course, that control simply can't exist without consent from the other person.

Now that many of the most popular misunderstandings of hypnosis have been further explained, that still leaves the question of, "If that's what hypnosis isn't, what *it is*?" In a scientific sense, hypnosis is actually very simple.

Because of the way that your brain functions is set up so that you can't truly multitask, you have to focus most of your attention on only one thing at a time. You may think you're a great multitasker, but you're only actively thinking about one of those tasks, two at the most on a good day. The rest of the stimuli coming in is quickly filtered to the back of the brain and left for when you're done with the task at hand. That excess information and excess weight all goes to your subconscious to be stored in the immediate memory, as it's going to be used very soon. The stimuli that aren't being fed to your conscious have to be pushed to the back, metaphorically speaking, as in your subconscious mind.

When we have a lot of information being filtered back to our subconscious, when we focus all of our attention onto one primary object or sensation, that's exactly when hypnosis can come into the equation. Someone in that exact state of intense focus is somehow very acutely lucid while not being very lucid at all, simultaneously. That sensation leaves you open to suggestion because you don't have the mental capacity to focus enough on that suggestion. Therefore, the suggestion is filed back into the subconscious. Because the conscious is the part of the mind that makes decisions, the subconscious has no real way of distinguishing what is "good" or "bad" information, it just keeps all information and organizes it for later, when we may or may not use it. Similarly, when you're listening to something separately while you browse the internet, you may find that you've accidentally started to type into the search bar what you're hearing, even if you didn't intend to. When we do things like this, we follow the suggestion because there's no part of our brain that advises against it. The brain trusts itself, so it follows all instruction it's given, no matter where it comes from, as long as the suggestion isn't outrageous or heinous enough to snap us out of that intense focus. Trance is simply the state of being so focused that you also become a little unfocused.

There are many ways that people react to being in trance. Some people tend to naturally forget whatever happens to them, or anything that's said, while in trance. Not many people have this acuity of memory loss, but it's not entirely rare for it to happen. Most subjects, however, tend to retain at least a large portion of their memory from the session, unless the hypnotist suggests otherwise. With no memory loss post-hypnotic suggestion, the subject will sometimes describe being in trance as a similar sensation to the small period of time when we're falling asleep; when we're still awake are relatively aware of our surroundings, but somehow a passive voyager in our own bodies. A subject in trance isn't asleep and they aren't comatose—but they aren't entirely awake either. The place between wakefulness and sleep is often considered where most ideal trance is. Some people in trance feel as though they were asleep, while some others may report feeling as though they were almost awake the entire time. This doesn't indicate anything about themselves or of the hypnotist necessarily—it only shows how diverse people's experiences can be. Having different experiences only allows beginning/novice subjects and hypnotists alike to widen their experience themselves, and allows them to become more comfortable with their partner and with different partners, they might each have in the future. Having more experiences in any space in life, including recreational hypnosis, is a good way to dispel any misconceptions you have about the practice. While many people perceive it as something that's malicious or a practice that seeks to control and manipulate others, it couldn't be farther from that. Hypnosis in any context serves to help people or to at least make an interesting and harmless party trick. This party trick, of course, can always be used to harm others. At this point, what was a cool and fascinating practice/hobby is now a tool that anyone can use poorly with the wrong intentions.

For example, it's a highly regarded rule of thumb not to hypnotize those who suffer from memory issues or chronic psychotic conditions. If you do put someone who falls into that category into a trance, the consequences of that decision can be disastrous for the subject—even in cases where the hypnotist is experienced and has put subjects similar into a trance before, every situation is different. So, no matter what, this situation can always be harmful. People with psychotic conditions can become much disoriented and even lash out, and a subject with memory problems may dissociate and lose part of their memory for a period of time, even if there was no suggestion to that effect. Of course, there are also hypnotists who use their abilities for malicious purposes and only use their skills to control others and manipulate them in a way that makes them uncomfortable or do something they may not want to do. Of course, a subject can only be made to do something they agreed to before, but their boundary may change, and the hypnotist in that relationship may not necessarily think of the best interest of the subject. To avoid situations like this, always make sure boundaries are clearly stated for every session. Also, it's important that the subject trusts his or her hypnotist every time a session begins. Without that trust, the subject can be made to feel uneasy even if that hypnotist does have good intentions.

Even with positive intentions, however, hypnosis isn't a state that everyone can enjoy for themselves. There are many people who don't enjoy the sensation of trance, often people who are afraid of losing control over themselves. Although this is a fear with no basis in truth as far as hypnosis is concerned, many people avoid hypnosis because of it and experience versatile reactions to trance when they do pursue it. This kind of reaction is usually not ever the fault of the hypnotist, but simply the result of fear and anxiety that exists not only in the conscious mind but in the subconscious as well. Many people have trauma that they try to either eliminate or further suppress with hypnosis—this can also cause very adverse reactions. Not only does it not often work, but the actual results can be fairly devastating to both the subject and hypnotist. There are some who suffer from memory issues or trauma who have their issues dealt with healthily via hypnosis—this is one of the many ways that hypnosis can help different kinds of people, and that help isn't a fluke. However, hypnosis can easily mess with memory in the long-term, as well as the perception of those memories and the ability to make new long-term memories in the present day. So, like you only go to a neurosurgeon for a very complicated procedure, only seek out very highly professional and experienced hypnotists who have a history of successfully helping people like you if you have a memory issue or one related to past traumas. The kind of memory loss experienced in trance, however, can also be solely helpful —some people have seen something they would much rather not remember. This something doesn't qualify as trauma; it was simply something unpleasant. Because whatever the thing or event was, wasn't necessarily traumatic or something long-term effect of the person's life or emotional state, it's something that can be much more easily dealt with. Going into a trance and having that memory blurred—as in hypnosis, memories aren't really being erased, exactly—is much less likely to harm the subject and is more likely to help them with no real added consequences. Of course, despite the much smaller risk, always seek out a professional when seeking out help for any kind of memory issue, no matter how small or how insignificant that memory may be.

Those insignificant memories can sometimes be lost in trance, depending on how deep it is. In the light trance, memory is almost always the exact same as before when the trance was induced. In a deeper trance, some of the details of memories may be muddy, but the overall picture stays the same as what it would have been before going into trance. The deeper the trance, however, the more time you may miss from a session and the more of the details may be completely gone. Even if memory loss isn't an effect otherwise induced within the session, it's a very common side effect of a deep trance. Like waking from a deep sleep, waking from trance may send a subject into a state of disorientation; this effect can be lessened if the trance is don't right, but it's difficult to completely eliminate. As a subject spends more time out of the trance, just like after sleep, more details come to them and they regain their memory. With trances that aren't particularly deep, the memory loss in the session will almost always return in a period of time. Of course, with particularly deep trances, the details will be much slower to return, and some of those details might not return. Of course, there are many cases in which every detail in intact after all trance, and this effect is really only caused when the trance is incredibly deep. Most novice or beginning hypnotists have a very hard time reaching this deep of a trance when they begin working with new subjects. It takes a very long time to be able to reach that deep of a trance, and many people that are able to reach it are people who understand the mild risk they may run. Don't try to ever deepen the trance "as much as possible", just to see how deep you and your subject can go—leaping into that hole can easily land you and your subject in a lot of trouble with trance, and possible a trance that the subject can't be woken up from without physical intervention. The effects are only mildly dangerous to the subject in the sense of their memories, but having a trance go too deep too son can have more severe effects on the subject emotionally, like any fear they may have had of not being able to control their trance has just been validated.

Trance is such an important part of hypnosis, both in that it's literally the biggest purpose of it and in that it's the part of hypnosis that helps others spiritually, emotionally, and physically. No matter what you may suffer from, there's a chance that hypnosis can likely help you recover from it and live a more satisfying life. Of course, it must be used in the hands of someone who knows what they're doing and knows how to do it right. If they're inexperienced or ill-intentioned, the results can be very dangerous. So, be careful who you trance with, and use the skill carefully.

Chapter Three:
We're All in Trance

We are all in trance very often, more than once a day. Up until hypnosis was introduced as a factor of modern medicine, it was treated as a ridiculous and magical way of treating illness, a placebo. However, when we daydream, we are in trance. When we are too caught up thinking while we drive and miss our exit, we are in trance as well. When we meditate, we are also in trance then. We are in trance so often in our lives that we don't notice it more often than we do notice it. If you're in the position of either a novice hypnotist or an experienced one, trance takes many different forms.

Trance is, put literally, just a heightened state of focus that every human goes into very often. When we feel overloaded with stress or sensation, when we feel exhausted, when we experience almost any change in our perception of the world, we go into at least a light state of trance. Many people associate trance with being overly vulnerable, suggestible, and easy to be manipulated. Because of the way hypnosis is often demonized in programming, especially children's programming, the understanding of what trance means is skewed. While trance is a state in which you are more open to suggestion, you don't lose a sense of identity or lose your will to be an individual. The "end result" of being hypnotized which is so often depicted in programming, and the state of trance itself, have little correlation. Trance is really only the first step in that process of relaxation; in which people get the idea that a subject in trance is a mindless slave open to whatever suggestion their hypnotist has for them. Nevertheless, many people fear either that they're too susceptible to trance or think they aren't susceptible at all. Neither of those things is true, but there are many things that can make a person more or less open to a hypnotic trance, like the following:

- Being more naturally intelligent – as mentioned in the previous chapter, contrary to popular belief, those who are less naturally intelligent are less susceptible to hypnosis. This is mainly because those individuals who are more highly intelligent are also more easily focused and more rational, which makes them much better candidates for hypnotic trance. This factor accounts less for the ability to recall information, as is so idealized in the most education system. Rather, the innate sense of awareness of the self, and awareness of others, play a larger role. Many people define intelligence as a measure of how open to taking in and absorbing information someone is, which goes hand in hand with the purpose of hypnosis.

- Being female – females are statistically more likely to be open to hypnosis than their male peers, simply because women tend to be more empathetic, less stubborn, and more focused. Additionally, women tend to be more open to stimulus and information is given to them by others. Being not necessarily submissive to everyone, but being much more able to take in suggestions and assimilate those suggestions into their own train of thought, allows for most women to be exceptionally skilled at going into trance.

- Being someone less prone to stubbornness – again, those who are more stubborn and less willing to listen to and compromise with others are also less likely to go into trance easily. However, there are many forms of scripts and inductions that are tailored to people who are more stubborn. Stubborn people also tend to be much more focused on their goals, so there's hope for them yet. However, more intelligent people sometimes tend to be more stubborn, perhaps due to awareness of their intelligence. So, it may be that all of those factors cancel out, leaving only the correlation between being less stubborn and being more open.

- Being extraverted – people who are more extraverted and outgoing also tend to be more empathetic and trusting, making them more suitable for hypnosis and trance. Although many stereotypical extraverts find it harder to focus on things, they are often more able to relax quickly and easily. On the flip side of this correlation however, more intelligent people tend to be more introverted, or at least less prone to putting themselves in stereotypical "party" scenarios.

- Being calm – obviously, being someone calm, patient, and relaxed makes you someone who fits the dream description for a novice or an expert hypnotist. Intelligent people tend to be more stubborn, but most highly intelligent people also tend to be calmer and more collected, always staying focused and keeping their head on straight. These attributes combined make for a very perceptive subject.

When someone goes into trance, there are many different things that can happen to them and their state of consciousness. Some people don't report really any change in their sense of consciousness, while others feel as though they fell asleep entirely. While the details of experiences range widely, there are many things that all proper trances have in common. For example, most people who go into trance correctly with a hypnotist who knows what he or she is doing reports feeling relaxed. Whether this is a purely physical sensation that leads to a mental sense of ease or vice versa, the sensation of relaxation is one that is vital to having a good hypnotic experience. Most people who experience trance also report feeling happy and refreshed afterward, something else that is very important when you first enter the field. Making your client or subject feel calm and relaxed, and overall positive, for the entire experience, is the key to improving their lifestyle and keeping them, either as a client or as a recreational partner. Being able to relax and let the details of the situation be handed over to your partner allows for the hypnotist to do their job more efficiently and makes the experience more positive for both parties.

Mental health and trance can sometimes interact in ways that are strange at best and highly dangerous at worst. Even with a subject and hypnotist who know and trust each other, and who have boundaries set clearly and distinctly, sometimes a person doesn't know even their own mind well enough to predict how it reacts to different things. Even if a person's conscious mind behaves a certain way, the subconscious may respond harshly to trance or suggestion. We often experience emotions that have no real reason or tether in reality. Similar to our intuition, which suggests what to do without giving any real "reason", sometimes we can feel scared and uncomfortable even though we have no reason to feel this way. This kind of anxiety can be triggered in some people by trance. If you're a hypnotist and you see this kind of reaction in your subject, bring them out of trance immediately and ask them if there is anything about their past experiences with hypnosis/mental health. Sometimes, there's nothing being hidden, but simply a deeply-seated reaction with no reason. If the subject and hypnotist both want to work through this psychological blockage, there are many ways to. If not, of course, it's unwise of any hypnotist to try and force a response, no matter their experience. If your subject expresses the desire to move past whatever subconscious blockages they might have, there are many ways you can help them. Here's how many hypnotists work with their subjects to move forward:

- Pinpointing what exactly elicits the unwanted response from the subject – if the subject is not comfortable going back into trance, tries to discover any words or phrases in particular that make the subject uncomfortable or anxious. If the subject is comfortable going back into trance, experiment with different kinds of inductions and approaches. If there are some specific words/ phrases that trigger the specific response, or a certain tone that makes the subject uncomfortable, evaluate if it's something you can change—that kind of language may make a lot of people uncomfortable.

- Working through the blockage – depending on the subject and on the blockage they experience, there are many different ways you could approach moving through it. If possible, it may be best to simply avoid the tone or phrases you use; sometimes we repress memories related to trauma, and a certain tone, phrase, or word can evoke memories or emotions associated with that trauma. However, if this isn't the case/the subject doesn't want to avoid the tone or phrase, there are ways to allow the subject to slowly get used to it. If the subject wants to slowly become acclimated to whatever makes them uncomfortable or anxious, it may be best to leave it alone for a short period of time. When the subject is ready, bring the word/phrase/tone into induction or casual conversation very briefly. After they become used to this kind of use, allow the phrase or tone to make its way more and more into the conversation, then into inductions and trance. After a while, the subject will find themselves much more used to the thing that once made them very uncomfortable, sad, or afraid. If the subject wants, some pairs may see fit to speed up that process, and simply continue the use of that tone or phrase as much as possible until the subject simply becomes accepting of it. Some situations don't allow for that kind of method— not all injuries are best healed with the bandage ripped off quickly. How to properly deal with this situation depends heavily both on the subject and on the matter that elicits the undesired reaction.

Trance is a very powerful weapon and one that must be used with good intentions. If a subject and a hypnotist don't have the same ideas about how a session should go, problems can occur because of this miscommunication. There are many ways to increase the effectiveness and efficiency of your trance by making sure you communicate clearly and safely with your partner. Understanding exactly what they want out of a certain experience will help both them and you, as a beginning hypnotist, to better map out induction and prepare for contingencies. But, this only accounts for trance when we're aware that we're in it. Since most people are in trance just about every day, how can a person be safe without knowing they're even in a form of trance?

The form of trance that most people go into doesn't actually trance in the way that it exists for hypnotists. For the sake of recreational hypnosis, trance is a state of being totally focused and relaxed, so that you take in the suggestion from the people around you. However, this isn't necessarily the working definition for everyone who experiences any kind of trance. The kind of trance we go into in our daily lives can be described as a very light waking trance. This kind of trance is one we go into most often, sometimes without even realizing we're doing it. When we read a book and begin to zone out from the world around us, too lost in the plot to pay attention to anything else, we're in a light trance. Even though we're still awake and alert and thinking, we aren't paying very close attention to anything else that might be going on around us. This light trance is completely harmless and is the same kind of trance we go into when we become lost in our thoughts while driving or daydream in class. The heavier the trance, the more likely that it's achieved more easily when induced by someone else.

Many people cling to the claim that "all hypnosis is self-hypnosis", maybe to comfort themselves when they feel afraid of losing control of themselves during a session. While, yes, the statement that all hypnosis is self-hypnosis isn't at all wrong, it isn't necessarily totally correct either.

You can easily hypnotize yourself to any degree that you wish. However, it can be difficult to get yourself to a certain place in trance without someone on the other end to guide you. This is why guided hypnosis is often so much more effective—when you're in a position where you have to both guide and be guided, you aren't allowing yourself to focus completely on that point of hypnotic focus. The trance can't reach as deep a state as many other trances you may find yourself in. However, self-hypnosis is a perfectly satisfying practice as well. It also eliminates the risk of having a rotten hypnotist who either doesn't know how to suit your needs/preferences or is genuine of malicious intent. Whatever the reason, some subjects don't like putting their trust in other hypnotists they may not know well, so they hypnotize themselves. This form of hypnosis is just as effective as guided hypnosis when done correctly. If you want to achieve a much deeper state of trance however, it's likely in your best interest to either seek out some other hypnotist to take your place or find resources online.

Those online resources can also technically count as "self-hypnosis" since whatever video or audio file you may play to induct yourself would never work without your consent. Of course, it can be hard to find the right file which suits your preferences or tastes. There's a massive spectrum of different hypnotists who work online, and whose effect can be felt without them being there in person. Many people seek out hypnotists that they can actually become friends with online. Hypnotizing someone over the phone, or even over text message, is possible with the right subject and hypnotist. Even though there's virtually nothing there to hold the induction together, it's the subject's willingness to continue and make ends meet psychologically to get the trance to "work", which makes the induction successful. It's the participation of the subject which makes those ends meet, which could be considered, in a way, hypnotizing yourself. That example then leads to blurring the lines between what is self-hypnosis and what is guided hypnosis, but the two states are the same if induced by different parties. The trance reached by the self and the trance reached by someone else, perhaps more experienced, are often the same at their core. Although different people bring different feelings, the sensation of trance doesn't change when you do it yourself. If you're in a position to be hypnotizing yourself, for whatever reason you desire to, there's no reason that your trance shouldn't be as satisfying as the same or similar trance induced by another hypnotist.

The sensation of trance can raise a lot of questions with some people once they become aware of what trance is and when they go into it. Some people become hesitant to zone off and daydream, sometimes since we demonize trance so much in some forms of media. Some people are simply afraid of losing the control they have over themselves. It's easy to feel scared by a mental space you don't entirely understand, especially when that mental space can sometimes make you feel as though you aren't thinking right. However, learning more about how you specifically go into trance can help you and many other people better understand yourself and understand hypnosis. If you're a hypnotist, pushing yourself to experience new people and experiment with different personalities can also help you gain more knowledge in the area you're pursuing. That understanding of trance is invaluable to anyone on either side of the induction. So, even just reading up all that you can on trances, different states of trance, and the potential effects of trance, can help you, in the long run, to be more successful as a hypnotist—after all, knowledge is power.

Chapter Four:
The Effect

You probably read or learned about the placebo effect at some point in school, but you may not have a deep understanding of what it is and how it applies to you.

The placebo effect is, in layman's terms, the effect of information on our brain, even though we have no actual change to back up the information. Think of two groups of people who are told that a pill they take will give them a headache. One of the groups is given an actual pill, which will actually induce a headache. The other group is given a sugar pill which has no effect on them physically and shouldn't The chances arc high that both parties will react negatively, with some degree of headache. Even though the second group was only given a sugar pill, they believed firmly that they would be given the same kind of pill as the other group. Because they believed they would have a headache, they had one. The powers of the mind are proven to have notably more effective than the powers of the body itself. This makes sense, considering the brain powers to the body and not the other way around.

Nevertheless, the placebo effect is large parts of the reason many hypnotic subjects who go into trance easily are not first-timers to the process.

Those who may be first-timers to the process may not be privy to what exactly is supposed to happen when their hypnotist begins trying to coax them into a trance. Because they have an idea that they should be doing something, the process itself is often not as effective as it can be. The ideal setting for someone who is just being introduced to hypnosis is that they are being hypnotized by someone they know and trust, and they are in a position to relax and trust the hypnotist to take care of the details. This way, the person can really focus is doesn't have their attention cluttered by what they should or shouldn't be doing.

On the other end of the spectrum, you have subjects who are veterans of the practice. Whether it is in the context of therapeutic hypnosis or recreational trance, those who have been hypnotized before finding it much easier to go into trance again. The more often they do it, the easier it becomes. In a way, the trance sticks with them and they find themselves able to relax and focus into one thing much easier and much faster than when their first time being hypnotized. Veteran hypnotic subjects often are much less hung up on details of what should happen and what to avoid. They know that trance is a fairly loose process that is mainly built off the emotions and the focus of two people, not the specific process of it. If you're a veteran hypnotist, therapeutic or otherwise, you also know well that the process of hypnosis is something that can mostly be done by yourself, so the presence of another person is only helping the process along. Therefore, how well that other person performs doesn't matter as much as new subjects/hypnotists often think.

If you're a first-time hypnotist or hypnotic subject, keep in mind that the other person may be nervous as well, if they're also new to the topic and the practice. Build off of each other's energy as you continue interacting until you find yourself in trance. While it's important to remain focused, making note of the "vibe" of the other person often helps majorly with keeping the session satisfactory for everyone involved. If the other person isn't nervous, take comfort in their confidence and let it lead you along. If you're a hypnotist, it's so important to be confident. Being able to sell the process, and sell yourself, to your subject is the best way to get them to believe in what you're doing and saying. If you're evidently unconfident, the subject will also feel unsure about what's happening, which can break the trance and cause both parties to leave the session feeling uncomfortable and unsure about their capabilities. Even if you feel unsure in your ability to succeed, the confidence is what will induce the placebo effect in your subject, at least to an extent. When you seem like you know what you're doing, the other person is going to believe more fervently that you do know what you're doing and is going to buy into it more. Believing that something is having an effect is almost the same as the actual physical effect, in many cases—including hypnosis, a process which mainly only takes the brain's cooperation to work.

Many native tribes in different parts of the world utilize the placebo effect, specifically for medicinal purposes. Think of all the home remedies, homeopathic healing, you've heard of or encountered. There are high chances that many of the people who grew up on those home healing remedies believe in them fervently. They believe in these kinds of home treatments because, to those who believe in their effectiveness, they really work. Even with no science, or evidence to back up the claims, the sensation of healing them likely experience is very real—this is the placebo effect at work. This same effect is the one that allows for novice hypnotists to get a head start when they first begin practicing their craft.

The adage "mind over matter" has always had more than a little skepticism from many people. However, the power of the mind takes its shape both in homeopathy and in hypnosis. The power of the mind in hypnosis is, in reality, what truly sells trance both as a product and an experience.

This is why so many people treat all hypnosis is self-hypnosis. A subject who is willing to understand the part they play in any induction is also a massive part of what makes the induction work at all. Many new subjects assume that when they look to be hypnotized, they're only looking for a moment to relax and zone out. However that isn't always the case—often, there are new hypnotists in hypnosis both online and in person, who need a subject's help to allow for the trance to actually work. Of course, the subject doesn't talk or put in much physical effort, but they help in that they allow for the hypnotist to do their job, and the subject fills in mentally for any mistakes the new hypnotist may make. This takes off a lot of pressure for both the hypnotist in question, and often for the subject as well—believing that the person on the other end knows exactly what they're doing allows the subject to focus on their job in that relationship, going into trance.

There are many ways that a subject can inadvertently help their hypnotist perform better, both for them and for any other subjects they may encounter in the future. Often, the way that a subject helps their hypnotist this way is unintentional, an employee of the placebo effect. Even though often the help a subject offers is usually unintentional, that help still goes a long way in making the experience better and more enjoyable.

For example, if a hypnotist is asking for a subject to relax and focus and breathe and whatnot, the subject's job is to focus intently on whatever the hypnotist asks. As a subject, allowing your mind to wander wherever it does unless otherwise requested of you by the hypnotist only makes their job harder. Many new subjects assume that being the subject is easy because you sit back and let the hypnotist take over everything. Except usually, the hypnotist doesn't know exactly how to take over things manually. Often, the subject must put in a helping hand and have their minds quieter than usual, be more focused than they might otherwise be so that the hypnotist has an easier job putting the subject into trance. Of course, the hypnotist is still the one guiding the subject. The hypnotist still calls the shots and builds up the induction and the trance. The only difference is that the subject is especially compliant. A subject going slightly out of their way to make the job of a novice hypnotist easier means that not only will the hypnotist have an easier time guiding the subject into trance, but that subject will also then get much more out of the experience, because they made it easier than it would have been for them if they had remained neutral.

Part of making a hypnotist's job easier is being able to use the placebo effect on yourself. Put simply, being able to trick yourself into focusing and relaxing, and responding positively to the requests and commands of the hypnotist, makes the experience better for both halves of the party. Being able to hypnotize yourself while also allowing the actual hypnotist to does their job as well, will always lead to a much more successful and much more satisfying state of trance. Of course, you aren't truly "hypnotizing yourself". While, to a degree, all hypnosis is partially self-hypnosis, there's no way for a subject to perform the entire ritual of hypnosis on their own to themselves without ruining some of the effects for themselves. While playing into the role of the subject more than you might need is very helpful to your hypnotist, it's also important to let them do their job as much as you do yours as their subject.

In the place of a hypnotist, you don't need to ask your subject to hypnotize themselves. If you're a beginner or feel very insecure in your abilities as of late, just try practicing on someone you know—ideally someone who's already very open to suggestion. Outwardly asking your subject to help you hypnotize them has almost the opposite effect as the subject helping of their own accord —because you asked them or help, you seem as though you're incompetent or not good enough to hypnotize them without their help. As they progress down into trance, the subject will likely begin to hypnotize themselves, if only just slightly. All you need is a little push from the placebo, and you're on your way to a subject who helps you hypnotize them without knowing. If you still want to bring up the idea or speed up the process of the placebo, simply try to buff up your inductions and scripts. Making them much more visually appealing, as well as appealing to the ear, will cause the subject to feel more comfortable. When a subject feels more comfortable, they're much more likely to play in their role as subject and allow themselves to go deeper, faster, than they might have gone into trance without any added descriptors or imagery. If not the first session, this trend becomes more and more stable with every session you have with that subject. That's the secret to the placebo effect, especially in hypnosis—the trick fails as soon as they know they're being tricked.

Obviously, the subject is not literally being tricked, as they consented beforehand. The line between playfully "tricking" your subject into helping hypnotize them and actually invading on their privacy is one that should be drawn hard. If you or your subject feel as though there may be some aspects of this session that makes them feel uncomfortable or as if they're being tricked, be honest with them immediately. There's no "upper hand" worth ruining the experience of trance for a subject. While honesty comes far before having some kind of advantage over them, if the subject is let in on the fact that you want their help to hypnotize them, you automatically seem a bit more unconvincing, and the trance might weaken before it had even begun. If they remain unaware, they mentally do the work before they mean to; they assume that you're confident if you seem confident, and seeming confident means seeming competent. Therefore, the subject wants to experience the trance to an even greater extent, and puts themselves further into a trance, helping you without even having to be asked. Of course, this doesn't necessarily work to such an extent on everyone. Some subjects don't help their hypnotists, and some subjects may teasingly resist hypnosis. This kind of resistance plays into another kind of induction and is not one meant for a first-time hypnotist. As a first-timer likely is still grasping the basics of how to hypnotize someone normally, someone outwardly resisting trance may overwhelm the hypnotist. However, this kind of subject is a semi-basic format of induction and only needs a little teasing in return. As a hypnotist, being uptight and anxious is not an option, no matter what kind of subject you have or what kind of induction you want to use. Another way the placebo effect has an impact on many hypnotists is not by influencing their subjects, but by directly influencing themselves. Many people cling to the "fake it 'til you make it" mantra, mainly because it usually works, to a degree.

If you're able to convince yourself that you're much more confident, much more competent, than you may believe otherwise, you'll act as such. Acting confident will both put the subject at ease and encourage them to participate in their own way in the induction. Eventually, your experience will have grown, and your confidence in your ability will now be much more real than you think. Still, practicing and starting out with friends or family is always a good first step, and a good way to begin building confidence sincerely. Being able to harness your confidence and your potential is the first step toward becoming a competent and skilled hypnotist, one who can tackle any kind of subject and any kind of situation. Being versatile and knowing how to deal with contingencies, keeping your cool no matter what, doesn't just convince your subject that you know what you're doing—in convinces you as well.

If anything, this is the true "trick" of the placebo effect—although often much weaker when used by someone who knows when it's working, the placebo effect works its "magic" on anyone and everyone. In the context of hypnosis, it can be a magnificent tool in closing the gap between preferences and can be a lifesaver when it comes to a subject that may be indecisive when it comes to a subject who may be particularly hard to please. To even a subject very easy to please, the correct use of the placebo effect, faking it until you make it, only increases how much that subject enjoys that particular trance, which reflects very well on you as a hypnotist. As a beginning, novice hypnotist, or as a professional or veteran to the scene, the placebo effect and being able to carry your charisma over gaps unfilled by experience or skill is an irreplaceable tool that can and will play a large and relevant role to your experiences in hypnosis.

Chapter Five:
Spectrum

We all respond differently to things. Our different reactions can be spurred by anything, really. Whether it is things that we've had to deal with in the past, things we have to deal with in the present, or something else entirely like genetics, we all have a certain affinity to different things. These things can be things like occupations we want, dreams we have, the fears we have. They can also take the shape of small things, like the different types of mannerisms we find attractive, and the different sounds we find the most pleasing to the ear. The lattermost of that list is what's most important when it comes to hypnosis. When coaxing someone to relax and into a trance, we have to use words that make them relaxed and focused. While, of course, you could always just use the words "relax", and "focus", those words become old and repetitive quickly, and show a lack of creativity. Of course, the tone is another very important aspect of hypnosis itself, but no tone can make up for a simply bland and boring induction. Getting down to the different sounds themselves which are most calming, like drawn-out vowels and softer consonants is what differentiates the novice from the veteran. Here's an example:

"Close your eyes and relax. Focus on one image in your mind, and relax. Relaxing more and more, focusing more and more until there's nothing left to focus on but the image in your head and my voice. Just keep relaxing and focusing."

While that induction is fine, and would likely work to an extent, it's repetitive and not very original. Also, it gives the subject two things to focus on at once and gives them no benchmark by which to relax or focus. You might be better off with something more detailed, like this:

"Close your eyes and breathe slowly, deeply, in and out. With each exhale, relax your body a bit more. Focusing on my voice a bit more with every breath out."

Even though that's shorter, it focuses more on what's important in any induction—that the subject understands clearly what's supposed to be happening. By giving them a benchmark by which to relax, with every exhale, they're able to actually focus without worrying that they're going too fast or too slow for the hypnotist. Although to an extent, more detailed is better, make sure that when you detail your induction, you focus the details on the part of the induction that is actually important to the purpose of the induction. For example, make sure that if you're going to add a lot of detail into something don't add the detail into breathing—add the detail into the feelings that come from breathing. Detailing breathing itself can also be fine, as long as the description lends itself to a calm and relaxed feeling. Adding more details to allow your subject to visualize the scenario better will allow them to do more of the work for you. Someone who is more adept at visualizing and losing themselves in a daydream or mental image is more able to be hypnotized and goes into trance more easily.

Some people like harsher sounds in their inductions, although generally more subjects prefer there to be softer and gentler words to their induction. Additionally, some people prefer their partner or hypnotherapist to be someone very professional and sure of themselves. Others prefer someone who is softer and more empathetic with them. This is up to the preferences of the individual, but whether those preferences are stated and understood or not can have a considerable impact on how well—or poorly—the session goes.

If you're a hypnotist with a subject who prefers the former type of hypnotist, who is more professional and even cold, make sure to keep your body and words in line with that preference. If you want to appear more professional and curter, speak short sentences that are succinct and get the point across. Make sure that when you approach and speak to the subject, you use a lower, more confident tone. Keep your posture more rigid than it may be otherwise, and it may help you to dress more professionally as well. If the subject prefers someone kinder and softer, make sure that your tone is quiet, but not in a way that makes you seem unconfident. The line between kind and weak-willed can be thin, but setting boundaries nonetheless and making your authority known helps make the distinction for everyone in the party. If you keep your voice quiet, soft, and comforting, that kind of subject will respond more positively. Many subjects seek out hypnosis as stress relief, so keeping your voice a tone that brings the subject peace and relaxation allows for that very process of stress relief to be more effective and efficient.

Some subjects don't respond very well to simpler inductions. Because of the "relax and focus" mantra can be worn out easily, a subject who isn't as much of a novice to hypnosis has likely already had experience with that exact mantra before, and want something more original. Like many things, a mantra loses its effect as it loses its novelty to the person it's used on. To mix things up a bit, try making sure that the hypnotic focus isn't always the same. If you keep the structure of the session the same—deliberate trance, no resistance or confusion-based sessions—you still easily have a few aspects of the sensation of trance that are open to manipulation and evolution. Changing your tone to fulfill a different vision the subject may have, or simply asking the subject to tether their focus to something else besides breath or their own bodies, are only some of those ways to change the set-up of the induction. Additionally, when you do change the hypnotic focus, it's also usually a good idea to then build the rest of the induction around that new point of focus. This may not be possible depending on what they focus is, but being creative and experimenting with what may or may not work for you and the subject is what allows for growth and for new, and better, experiences.

For instance, one of my personal favorite beginner's inductions centers on a flame. It doesn't necessarily require any kind of resistance, but that aspect is open to whoever utilizes that template. The base of that induction usually goes something like this:

"Focus on the candle's flame. Burn the image of its flame into your head, so that you can envision it perfectly even when you close your eyes. This flame is your mind, your focus, your consciousness. It flickers and sways, back and forth, left and right, never still and never stagnant. It can be strong and versatile, hard to snuff out. Focusing on that flame, on your will and your mind, so strong and hard to budge. The flame is your mind. Your mind is the flame. Imagine the words, reading over and over in your mind, the flame. The flame is your mind. The more you stare at the flame, the fewer thoughts cloud your focus on the flame, on your mind. The less distracted your mind becomes, the more you can focus on the flame, your mind, the flame."

Repetitive, but how repetitive is up to the person using it. After the hypnotist deems that the subject is deeply entranced by the flame and makes a strong subconscious association between the flame and their conscious mind, there are a number of things you can do. Moving the flame out of view of the subject, or simply obscuring the subject's vision, makes for a good sharp transition from something very clear to focus on, to nothing at all. Revoking that object of focus leaves the subject very focused and relaxed, but no longer has the objective of keeping their eyes open or focusing directly on that flame. You could also count down, as many hypnotists do. The transition from something to focus on to nothing to focus on can be too sharp for the subject and can make them disoriented. This breaks the trance and cancels out the effect of that flame, so detailing what's going to happen to the subject and then counting down to that result allows for a smoother transition from waking trance to non-waking trance. Many hypnotists may completely snuff out the flame once the countdown ends, keeping the association between the subject's mind and the flame strong, and allowing for the subject to fall into a non-waking trance. A countdown of that nature may look something like this;

"I'm going to count down from 5 to 0. When I reach 0, your mind, the flame, will be gone. No thinking, no thoughts, gone with the wind, the flame. 5, falling deeper and deeper; 4, the flame, your mind, swaying and rocking and almost going out, your mind; 3, closer to smoke and nothing, no thinking; 2, the flame, your mind, bending and so far away; 1, on the edge of smoke and no thinking, so far away and 0."

This template is subject to change and something to be added to. However, keep in mind that what you choose to change about how these templates are worded may reflect negatively within your sessions. Taking the time to understand what's best for you and for your subject is the only thing that will always yield the most ideal outcome. You may choose not to add a countdown—however, if you do, the "0" should be followed immediately with snuffing out the candle or otherwise inducing a non-waking state of trance. The swift transition between waking trance and non-waking trance tends to be softened when accompanied by a sort of countdown since it lays out clear instruction and clarification for the subject. Therefore, the trance is much less likely to be broken by that transition.

When a subject moves from a waking trance to a non-waking trance, nothing much actually happens internally. All that really goes on between those two states of mind is that the slow, sluggish train of thought finally comes to a complete halt. Some subjects have stopped that train of thought while still in a waking trance, however, depending on how deep that trance was. We often think of non-waking trances as much deeper than waking trances, and those kinds of trances are generally not as responsive. When in a non-waking trance, a subject is much less likely to respond to a suggestion or command verbally. The subconscious is incomplete or almost complete control of the mind at this point and from here on out, the subject is less likely to remember details of the session. This isn't the case for all subjects, but it's the general case for most.

The non-waking trance is also generally where the deepest parts of the psyche are explored in clinical hypnotherapy. When the subconscious has that much of a hold on a subject, they have lowered inhibitions and are much more likely to respond honestly to a question, although some subjects may answer incoherently. Because that deeper, non-waking trance is more like sleep than a waking trance, the subject may feel more rested afterward from this part of the induction than in the transition into waking trance. When the subject responds—if they respond—they may answer in a slurred voice or in a way that is otherwise inappropriate for that person. Their subconscious allows them to speak "freely", which may be a new kind of persona for them to show to other people. They may hide that persona on purpose because they feel ashamed of the way they can sometimes act behind closed doors. Or, the subconscious may simply be finding a way to manifest itself more clearly. This disparity in behavior isn't found in all subjects, but it is found in many—the disparity between the behaviors of the subject and how they behave in a very deep trance can also be found more acutely in people who suffer from disorders like schizophrenia or Dissociative Identity Disorder, more popularly known as Multiple Personality Disorder. When someone with a disorder which can cause a serious difference in their behavior, and which also might affect their memories, may be difficult to deal with for a novice hypnotist. What may seem to some like a normal shift in personality may actually be a dissociative episode for someone who suffers from a disorder. Be careful with your subject and make sure that wherever you are, you and your subject are both in a place that is healthy and safe. It may also be in your best interest to have someone else within the space, such as someone the subject knows and trusts—after all, you don't have to have a dissociative disorder or a history of dissociative episodes to have one now. Being at risk for one or more of these dangerous possible side effects can endanger both you, as a subject, and the hypnotist. Being able to control yourself and being open to hypnosis are things which may collide every now and then, but many people are not so at the risk that they can't take care of themselves when they do suffer from a dangerous side effect.

There are more subtle ways that your subject may have an adverse reaction to something you and them try out within a session, and the results are not always predictable, or positive. The key to being able to gain as much experience as you can, both as a hypnotic subject and as a hypnotist, is experimentation—namely, experimenting as safely as possible. Some partners within recreational hypnosis have a kind of safe word—some more clinical relationships do as well. Having a word or phrase that a subject can tether onto in case they suddenly feel uncomfortable, unsafe, or simply feel as though they're having a negative or adverse reaction to something you may have been experimenting with. Communication is important in any kind of relationship, even ones that are strictly platonic or strictly professional. Being able to communicate when something may have gone wrong or even if nothing has gone wrong, will ensure that the encounter is more satisfying for both people.

While the placebo effect is something strong, and something that can help many people overcomes their fears, it isn't something that you should ever substitute for consent or for safety. If you feel unsafe or scared, even if you know it isn't a rational fear, tricking yourself into thinking you're not in danger can become a very troublesome habit that can later turn into something which threatens your state of mind. Both for a subject and a hypnotist, the placebo effect is a strong thing which can allow you to be more confident and more adaptable; it is not something that switches out for real peace of mind. Even in the case of building one's own confidence, a way that the placebo effect is meant to be used, the placebo effect is essentially worthless without the use of methods which actually build up your confidence. The placebo effect works best as a temporary crutch, not something that replaces confidence totally—a person who uses the effect to build up their self-esteem but does nothing to actually better that confidence will never be truly confident, they'll only ever end up seeming delusional to others. The placebo effect is an important tool for anything diving into hypnosis and anyone who's experienced in the field. It's a massive part of the language of hypnosis, and will always play a large role in how hypnosis evolves, as is the way that individuals of all different kinds respond to different situations in the context of hypnosis.

Chapter Six:
Script-Master

Being able to construct your own script is an integral part of making it as a hypnotist. Not only is being creative an important part of building your own induction script but knowing what you subject specifically would like and what wording/attitude would make the experience best for them is also massively important. Some subjects prefer longer and more detailed scripts, while some other subjects can fall into trance with a fairly short, brief prompting. Often, the more experienced a subject is, the more they're able to fall into trance efficiently and stay in trance more effectively. For the sake of both novice hypnotists and hypnotists who aren't very confident in their capabilities, the ability to confidently build an induction or script is very relevant to keeping a partner or client coming back to you. In addition, it's in your best interest as a beginning hypnotist to quickly develop the ability to gauge what kind of induction a certain person may be more drawn toward. Of course, the kind of induction you use pertains more to the recreational than the clinical.

The way that your scripts flow depends heavily on what kind of subject you're dealing with. If you know that the person you're going to hypnotize is nervous about their first time in a trance, or you know that the person is often anxious in general, you may want to give them a simpler first script that is not only very easy to follow but very relaxing. Overall, your scripts should be easy to follow and calming, but pay particular attention to those details of the script when the subject at hand is either very nervous, sensitive, or new. This kind of script not only calms the nerves of that subject, but it also eases them into the idea of hypnosis is falling into trance. If you have a subject who is more confident, or even someone who is looking for a challenge, you may then want to take a very different route. If you have a subject who either doubts your abilities or simply doubts that they can be hypnotized— this is in the case that these expressed sentiments by the subject are coy and playful, not genuinely malicious or meant to be harmful--you may want to go in the direction of resistance induction. However, a resistance induction is not exactly the best map to follow when it comes to easing your way into hypnosis—resistance-based subjects and inductions are often more suited toward more experienced hypnotists. However, if you want to learn how to perform one easily, it's not massively difficult either.

A resistance induction is a very different kind of script that doesn't necessarily focus on relaxation and being calm right out of the gate. This is because often when a subject is trying to resist attempts at hypnosis, they will go out of their way to stay tense and to not listen. In a sense, you have to trick someone like this in order for them to "lose" the challenge that they've set for themselves. Of course, never perform any kind of induction, even a resistance induction, on someone who has not previously consented for you to try to hypnotize them.

The difference between a resistance prompt and any other kind of induction is that instead of the power being anchored to the physical—being relaxed and focused leaves the body less reactive, more vulnerable, and more open to suggestion—the power is anchored completely to the psychological state of the person you're looking to hypnotize. For example, the person who is trying to resist a hypnotic state is not going to relax, or breathe deeply. They are going to do the exact opposite of what you request of them. Although to a beginning hypnotist, this seems very troublesome, there are a few things you can do to wear down the stubbornness of a subject who feels challenged by your attempts, or your confidence.

Something crucial about subjects like this, who take on this "challenge" --there is what some consider two types of subjects who you use a resistance induction on. There is the first type, the kind of subject who genuinely feels more than a little threatened by the idea that they can be "controlled". Of course, they aren't really being controlled, but the threat appears just as intimidating to most people nonetheless. They don't want to feel as though they've lost control and want to prove it to themselves and others that they're strong-willed. The downfall of this type of subject is that hypnosis isn't really a battle of willpower at all. It's a battle of focus. Anyone can be hypnotized. The only way to truly evade being hypnotized by anyone at any time is by plainly refusing to listen to anything they have to say. Cutting off any visual or auditory contact with that person is the thing that will guarantee a person is "safe" from that hypnotist, and at no risk of falling into trance. However, that's just the thing about coy subjects like that—because they consented previously to the entire experience, they obviously do want to be hypnotized, or at least want to participate in a kind of "struggle". Often, subjects that make a kind of game of resisting think of it as just that, a fun game for them to play. There's no malicious intent behind it, an often no real fear either. No, it's often simply a matter of being coy and enjoying the fight for dominance. The key to "winning" against subjects like this is to be consistent in how you approach them verbally. Never faltering and letting them know non-verbally that you have no intention of backing down from your battle of will, being consistently confident, is enough to let them know that there's no way for them to win. A battle of resistance often isn't really one that centers on the actual strength of will or experience—it's about two things, really; consistency, and charisma.

Consistency is more obvious—if you don't give in to their coy behavior, they have no choice but to either keep "battling" or to give in to the hypnotist, who has them beat in mental stamina. Being able to keep up your defenses longer, simply mentally outlasting them is enough on its own usually. However, sometimes you also need to do a bit of convincing—rather, proving to them that you have the upper hand, not only in will power but in pure psychology as well.

Anyone who willingly consents to be a hypnotic subject wants to be hypnotized. That's the fact of the matter, and there's absolutely no shame in hiding it. That's the other thing about more subjects who choose to act coyer about the session—they're often embarrassed by their want to be hypnotized, so they may act out as if that's the very opposite of what they want. Being confident enough to point out the obvious without being intrusive or predatory will open up the floor for the subject to understand exactly what's going on, and how to go forward from there. Of course, they likely won't immediately concede—if they did, that game would no longer be any fun for them or for their hypnotist. So, understand where the boundary lies between what is reciprocating that coy attitude, and what is infringing on the consent of the subject. Of course, that line shouldn't be very thin, to begin with, but the boundary was set as it was between the hypnotist and subject for a good reason. Namely, being able to distinguish what is "too much" for that particular subject.

Again, most beginning subjects won't be so coy, and may just be unsure about the entire situation. If they don't feel comfortable and seem unsure when prompted for consent, they likely aren't in a good place to consent to that kind of act. So, let them go. They aren't a viable subject if they aren't 100%, totally willing to engage in the session as much as possible. Any uncertainty means "no", just as much as plainly saying "no". This is the best way to make sure you avoid an adverse reaction, such as an anxiety attack.

Building your own inductions build your confidence as a hypnotist, and allow for more ideas, more creativity, as a hypnotist to flow as well. Simply finding your scripts online all the time and not being able to manufacture your own makes for a boring and bland writer that doesn't know how to appease their audience. If you want to be able to better write your own scripts, try some of these tips:

- Understand how you speak, in a hypnotic context – the idea of building your own hypnotic voice will be covered in the next chapter, but for now, be able to listen to yourself speak in your earliest sessions and build off of that. It shouldn't be incredibly hard to analyze your speech patterns but note the ways your intonation changes when you speak to a subject in trance. The ways that your voice changes are the same ways that you should speak in any script you write, so be able to write your scripts accordingly. Understanding how you speak normally, and how you speak to a subject in the context of hypnosis, allows you to have a better grasp of what exactly you want to get across to your subject. Ask any of the subjects you've dealt with in the past any impressions they get from the way you've spoken to them. Based on their responses, note any disparity between the idea they understand and the idea you're trying to convey. For example, a hypnotist might think his hypnotic voice is very professional, while his subjects may feel intimidated and even threatened by his tone of voice. Based on the general consensus of the responses, the hypnotist changes his hypnotic scripts and the way he speaks to better fit the idea that he wants to convey; professionalism. Being able to pick up on ways to clarify your points and intentions when speaking to a subject in trance is especially important since the subconscious mind takes essentially all instruction at face value. This refers to both the literal wording that the hypnotist might use, as well as their intonation. Even if you say the words you want to, saying those words the wrong way may upset the subject, or confuse them. Be as clear as possible with both your inductions and your instructions. Saying "focus and relax" gets the point across bluntly and saves time, but it doesn't give the subject very clear instructions. Instead, saying "focus on (object or sensation) and relax as you (breathe deeply/close your eyes/etc.) offers much more detailed instruction and lets the subject know that you have a clear idea of what you want them to do. Even to the subconscious, this difference can mean the world, even though you sacrifice a small bit of time for it. Channeling that amount of specific detail into your scripts and inductions will also mean a world of difference, no matter what kind of induction it is or what kind of subject you're working with.

• Although detail is important, still stay to the point – if you wander off verbally for too long or get onto tangents, the subject is more likely to subconsciously become distracted, and the trance may weaken or even break. Although it's massively important to specify instruction and what you want from the subject, it's also important to stay directly on the topic of whatever the induction may be about. If you're dealing with an induction that allows the subject to fantasize something very specific, don't ruin that fantasy by moving off into a different or shifted fantasy. Not only does this break focus on the subject, but it also makes it much easier for them to become confused. Too many instructions at once cause a lot of problems, but detailing only a few makes the experience more immersive for both the subject and their hypnotist. Finding that middle ground between a creative script and a scatter-brained one makes it much easier for the subject to follow along with the induction and feel as though they're included in that fantasy, whatever it may be about.

- Always ask for feedback from the subject – once out of the trance, make sure that you ask them shortly after what they thought specifically; what details they really enjoyed, and what aspects of the session they might change if your roles were switched. Of course, some of the feedback is going to be up to the subject's preference and shouldn't all be taken as indicative of the vast majority. However, it's important to get a general idea both for the sake of working again with that subject in particular and asking a wide range of subjects—even ones that you personally haven't worked with—what they've thought about different approaches and different tactics in their experience. You may be surprised by what you find, and whatever you find out about the vast majority of subjects you encounter may also tell you something that you can improve upon for yourself. Whatever you change, however, be sure that whatever subject you're currently dealing with is alright with whatever content those changes guarantee. It can be very difficult to discern what's good for a certain subject and what isn't--always be careful about where boundaries lie and whether or not they change when you do decide to make changes to your approach.

As always, the most important thing about building your own script is being able to stick to something you want, and being able to stay true to yourself and how you speak personally. If you take on a certain persona while building up your hypnotic voice, that's perfectly fine, and normal, as long as you make sure that the persona you build doesn't take over who you really are. It's that personality beneath the persona that actually makes up the scripts, and it's the more important part of who you are as a hypnotist. Trying to destroy the individuality of your own personality and just building up a script that you think is the best objectively, is always much more exhausting than simply being true to yourself and writing what makes you feel the best about your ability. Writing a script and being able to creatively come up with new approaches to different kinds of people is what makes or breaks a new hypnotist, whether they can do it consistently or not. If you feel comfortable enough with your capabilities to consult with the people around you and build up your own storylines for your subject, you already have the mechanisms of a fantastic hypnotist. A hypnotist who is able to be creative, which sets you apart from the majority of the other hypnotists entering the field. We often become so lost in how cool hypnosis can look, and feeling of it, that we often forget the work that has to go into it to make the experience the best it can possibly be.

Chapter Seven:
How To Build A Voice

Being able to build your very own, personalized hypnotic voice is an important part of making the experience with recreational hypnosis unique to both parties within that session. The hypnotic voice often becomes a part of the hypnotist's persona when they get into hypnosis. The effect that their voice has on different subjects will range from person to person, so the voice will change slightly sometimes to better fit the subject. However, the ideal hypnotic voice is one that doesn't need to be changed an incredible amount to do the job for as many hypnotic subjects as possible. That's generally the main goal for any hypnotist trying to enter the field of hypnosis and be successful—to be able to cater to as wide an audience as possible shows not only that you can be a capable hypnotist, but a flexible one as well.

Think about how your normal voice sounds to other people. There are some voices which have the qualities needed for ideal hypnosis already. Most voices don't—there's something dull, or obnoxious, or grating about the voice. Every single voice, however, can be influenced and improved upon to achieve the ideal result of a good hypnotic voice. The point of having a good hypnotic voice is, firstly, to be able to persuade others and to have a positive effect on those around you. Secondly, having a good hypnotic voice saves the hypnotist an enormous amount of trouble when putting a subject into trance.

As the goal of the first part of trance is finding a way for the subject to focus and relax, having a voice that is easy to listen to but not so that it takes up the entire subject's attention, is ideal. When the hypnotist has a very pleasing voice—one that's calm and softer, more droning—the subject is more easily swayed to relax and focus. However, the subject shouldn't actually be focusing on the hypnotist words (unless otherwise specified by that hypnotist). The wording of the hypnotist's script isn't usually very important past the initial instruction—after being told to focus, relax, close the eyes, take heavy and slow breaths, and so on and so forth, the instruction becomes repetitive and the subject often loses some of the interest in what exactly they're saying—and the sound of the hypnotist's voice alone is what carries the subject's relaxation for a lot of the remainder of the session. Additionally, the hypnotic focus of the subject usually isn't the hypnotist's voice. If it is, it often serves as a secondary focus or a tether. Often, subjects are instructed, or choose, to focus their attention on blinking, breathing, or some stationary fixture in their environment. This often serves them well; so many subjects don't rely on the words of the hypnotist too much.

However, even if you don't focus on the words of a person speaking to you, you still register their voice on some level. Although you don't pay attention to what you hear, you still hear it. When you don't pay attention to the specifics, those details quietly slip past the conscious mind and into the subconscious, where they take a much deeper hold on the subject. It's there, in the subconscious, taking deep root so that the suggestion can influence you in trance. Although that may sound scary, it's a normal part of the subconscious and it happens to us every time we hear background noise during our daily lives. Conversations we hear from others in the background of our daily activities worm their way into our subconscious mind and influence us slightly, whether we know it or not. The subconscious mind still has safeguards that prevent us from doing something ridiculous or harmful, because the conscious mind still functions most of the time, even when things slip into the backs of our heads. We're usually just pretty good at focusing and not letting ourselves be distracted by that background noise—after all, most scientists agree that if the brain paid attention to every single piece of stimulus it received, it would've long exploded by now.

That noise, whatever it may be, might be something that can qualify as hypnotic—like white noise generators or looping videos of rain sounds. They're soft and droning noises with little to no variation to their sound over long periods of time. Therefore, much like the "proper" hypnotic voice, they're easy to focus on loosely, while being able to relax while the sound filters down to our subconscious. It's easy to listen to sounds like that since they're so droning. Because they're boring, we find ourselves relaxed by them, and often don't even realize it when we do slip away into a kind of waking trance. That kind of trance is light and very easy to break, but a deeper state of trance is achieved by the same methods. That's why usually; a hypnosis audio file will have some kind of droning noise in the background. Whether it be white noise, binaural audio, or some other kind of soft and, quite frankly, boring sound, the background music is what calms us without us even knowing it. If we only had the sound of a voice in the background, there would be something inherently unnerving about the sound, or lack thereof.

To analyze your voice is to be able to better understand the effect you can have on your subject. Most voices aren't naturally fit for the ideal hypnotist's sound, so a lot of people new to hypnosis feel discouraged by the idea of their voice not being fit for the field. While those individuals with voices naturally fit for it have a natural advantage over some of their peers, it's far from impossible to improve upon your voice to make it more suitable for your subject. While there's a certain sound to a hypnotist that automatically makes them more generally appealing to the vast majority of subjects, almost all subjects you encounter will have a slightly different idea of what a hypnotist's voice would ideally sound like. While everyone has their niches, here are a few of the more general things that many people seek out in the voice of a partner, inside of and outside of hypnosis.

- Generally, subjects enjoy a lower voice, softer voice—a voice that's sultrier, even if not in a romantic sense, is any subject's perfect idea of the perfect sound. Not every subject likes a lower, deeper voice, but most people find that kind of tone alluring, if not plainly attractive. Even in the case of a female hypnotist, most subjects enjoy a hypnotist who has a much lower vocal register. If you want to lower your voice or make it deeper to make your sound more alluring, try keeping your head lower when you speak. The main point of lowering your voice is to make you sound less anxious and more confident. Someone who's anxious about what they're doing raises automatic suspicion with the subject—if they don't know what they're doing and trust their skills, why should their subject? So, however, you see fit to calm yourself down and relax your body/voice, make sure that however you do it involves relaxing your body in some way. A lot of the reason we may sound anxious at times is that we tend to instinctually pitch our chins up. Notice whenever you watch a singer try to hit a note that might be too high for them, their jaw may start to drift upward. When we raise our chins higher, our vocal cords become slightly more strained and we make higher sounds. Although this works well if you're trying to achieve a higher sound, it's also not healthy for your throat, and seriously strains your vocal cords. When we lower our heads, people generally have a much lower, gruffer sound to their voice. Also, releasing all the tension from your body, especially around your chest and shoulders, will help your vocal cords to relax the following suit. With your entire body more relaxed, you find yourself less likely to raise your chin up and speak anxiously. As for speaking quietly and softer, that can be more up to word choice than a physical change to your speaking. Speaking slower is generally more attractive to subjects because it makes the hypnotist seem more confident, more charismatic, and more caring. Speaking slower and softer also makes for a much more droning sound, a boring noise that's more likely to lull the subject into a trance with ease. Taking care to build the habit of speaking slowly, softly, keeping your chin lower, and making sure to keep an even tone are very small details on the surface, but they can make a massive difference in how effective your hypnotic voice is.

- Some subjects like a colder voice, some like a warmer tone—this varies a significant amount from subject to subject, although many subjects you encounter will prefer a hypnotist with a very warm voice. This is an easy change to make for most, but some people have a very professional tone without intending to. If you're in a position where you want to try and change the way your voice sounds to fit the preferences of your subject, try lowering your voice when you speak to the subject. Even being quieter can make your voice sound calmer and softer if the actual words being spoken are the exact same. If you want a colder voice, be sure to speak a bit louder, with less of an even tone. Don't shout or speak in a way that breaks the subject's trance, but adding a sharper sound to some of your words gives off a colder and more professional energy. Some subjects really enjoy a hypnotist who speaks that way, as it portrays a certain level of calm confidence. However, many subjects instead prefer a softer voice as it portrays more empathy, and makes them feel more comfortable, safer.

Certain words also affect the way that we sound to different people. Everyone has different experiences that shape how they perceive different people and details, so one subject may see your voice as calm and collected, while another subject may actually feel threatened, in a sense, by the colder and more professional aspect to your tone. Even choosing to use different words without changing much about the way you say those words can have a massive impact on how you're perceived by your subject. For example, an induction that begins like this, using the "flame" induction from earlier:

"Focusing on the fire, and calming down with every breath, every breathes bringing you farther and farther down and more relaxed..."

Is perfectly fine and gets the job done, but it may feel too professional to some subjects. In a sense, a hypnotic induction is almost like poetry, in that the sound of the words coming from the hypnotist make up how the audience—the subject—will respond to those sounds. Trying a beginning more along these lines;

"Focusing gently on the flame, flickering with every soft exhale you take, every deep inhale. Relaxing with the small flame, quiet and softly swaying, back and forth..."

Focuses a lot more on details—using alliteration and softer adjectives allows for the subject to have a better idea of both whatever you're trying to get them to visualize, and makes that subject feel safer and much more at peace— that is, if that subject takes more to a hypnotist with a softer and gentler voice. To have a more poetic take on an induction generally really helps with writing your own induction which has a positive effect on your subject, more poetic writing leading to gentler and more comforting words—or colder and calmer sound, if that's what that specific subject has more of an affinity toward. Being able to use more imagery in your induction can make the difference between a satisfies subject and a subject who leaves feeling uncomfortable—that imagery is what shifts based on the knowledge that you have on your subject's preferences, to better suit them and make them feel personally much safer and more secure with you as their hypnotist. Personalizing things can mean so incredibly much to some people.

It can be hard to cater to every subject you come across, but both gaining more of an understanding of their preferences as a subject and learning to slightly change your persona with the subject you work with—as long as that shift stays within your boundaries—can help both you as a hypnotist gain experience, and help the subject feel more at peace with you as a partner. Generally speaking, the ability to be flexible and change your style for the subject you interact with is a sign that the hypnotist isn't rigid, meaning they can work with just about any different subject, really any personality type. That flexibility and ability to adapt is precisely what will put you ahead of the curve, as far as new hypnotists are concerned. The ability to grow and adapt is important in both any kind of work environment and any hobby; so whether you're looking to become a hypnotist to put bread on the table, or to simply find a space where you can have fun and enjoy yourself while meeting new people, being able to adapt to new people and a diverse range of those new people, makes moving forward in your journey a lot easier.

Chapter Eight:
The Rising Action

Such a massive amount goes into putting a subject into a trance, keeping a subject in trance, and making sure that the trance is satisfying. However, not a lot often goes into whether or not the subject is carefully woken up from that trance. As touched on in past chapters, there are many adverse and dangerous reactions that can result if a subject is not taken proper care of throughout the entirety of their session. Not only do they run the risk of serious health effects such as intense bouts of anxiety or memory loss, but there's a much higher risk that they can wake up disoriented and uncomfortable. Of course, that result's incredibly preferable compared to that of a dissociative episode, but it still definitely isn't a very pleasant thing to have to deal with after a supposedly relaxing and calming experience. There are a lot of general rules of thumb when it comes to taking care of your subject as you come out of the trance and after waking up from the trance. In general, thinking of a person in a deep trance the same way you consider a person you see sleepwalking sets up a good template to follow.

Much like a sleepwalker, you should never, ever, wake up someone who's in deep trance physically or suddenly. The sudden jolt can immediately take them out of whatever relaxed state they had just happened to be in, and they may lash out at you, if only for having to take a moment to process now being awake. Instead, lead them back up the way that you would lead them down into trance. This can be with a countdown or without one, it doesn't particularly matter exactly how you go about making the transition up gentle, as long as you do make it gentle. Waking up a subject with a countdown might look something like this:

"(After fulfilling all that you had intended for that session) ...And now, we're going to count back up from 1 to 3, and when I reach 3, your eyes will open. Refreshed, relaxed, satisfied, happier. From 1, feeling your thoughts stirring and your mind shifting, rising up and up. 2, the world around you coming back into focus and my words much clearer now, more awake and aware. To 3, awake and eyes open."

In most all situations, something similar to that should do the job in waking up your subject and allowing them a moment to get comfortable with where they are and allowing for them to process the last period of time in which they were in trance. It can take a few moments, so don't immediately prompt or bombard them with questions or asking for feedback. Instead, ask simple questions, like "How do you feel?" and allow them a few moments to articulate their thoughts and answer coherently. Afterward, if you feel the situation is appropriate, strike up a more passive conversation with them and allow them to answer at their own pace. Giving them space and time they likely need to process their returning surroundings helps them feel more comfortable with you, as well. Depending on how deep the trance was or how used to trance that subject is, they may or may not need more or less time to get back to their normal functioning self—be patient.

However, there are some subjects who don't wake up from trance the first time you try to initiate it. This can be alarming at first, but don't lose your calm when it happens, and don't immediately resort to shaking them and otherwise disturbing them. If they don't respond immediately, they may be taking a minute to wake up. If, however, they don't wake after a minute or two, begin prompting them with questions as if they were still in trance. Ask them simple things that don't require much thought at all-- "yes" or "no" questions are always best. If they respond to those questions, simply try the countdown again, or some other method of slowly waking them up. If the subject doesn't respond to any prompting, or their name being called, it's likely time to interfere physically. Don't be concerned, however, since the most likely cause is the subject just falling asleep. Although it can be embarrassing for first-time subjects, and not something that they may be proud of admitting, it's nothing to be ashamed of and it doesn't indicate anything wrong with the subject physically or psychologically. When woken up, still be as gentle as possible, trying not to yell their name or prompt them more violently than necessary. After they've woken up, give them room and time to process being woken up. They may jolt awake and wonder where they are, but answer them calmly and let their memory come back to them naturally. It can be an embarrassing but fairly frequent occurrence, especially for new hypnotists and subjects, to have a session where the subject falls asleep in the middle of trance. It doesn't necessarily mean that the hypnotist was boring by any means—it just means that maybe the subject was tired, or got a little too comfortable. They relaxed but didn't focus enough to keep themselves awake. Because trance is considered by most as compared to the mental space between being awake a being sleep, finding that middle ground perfectly every time can be asking a bit too much from a new subject. Not only that, but there are other embarrassing and laughable mishaps that can happen with those new to hypnosis. Often, a subject may respond in a ridiculous way—imagine being prompted "think about your favorite thing in the world...", and the subject slowly responding, "Donuts..."--or the hypnotist may lose their confidence. It's alright to experiment and fail every now and then as a new hypnotist, and it's alright to "mess up" at first as a new subject. It can be really difficult to find exactly what feels the best for you and your partner, so try not to feel bad if you find you and your partner end up in a situation that makes you feel ridiculous at first—it's those exact situations which make hypnosis so fun, laughing at those exact situations once you look back at them again.

After your subject has woken up and taken the time they need to recover their thoughts, feel free to ask them any questions about the session they might have, or any feedback. The feedback you receive can help you later on as you move from subject to subject. Anything the subject feels could have been better about the session, or anything they feel was really good and/or interesting about the session, make note of for the future! If and when you have a session with a different subject, that advice and praise may come in handy, either to solidify your confidence or to improve upon the last session you had. Although all subjects will be different, there's a high chance there will be a correlation between what one subject likes and doesn't like and the likes and dislikes of another subject. Even if not, there's usually a group of subjects which likes the same things as one of the other subjects you've had in the past. No matter how niches the interests or preferences of that specific subject may be, you just might encounter someone else in the future with the same niche interests.

Aftercare is an important part of any relationship, even if the context of the hypnotic session is totally platonic. Ask the subject if they want anything, and have a conversation about anything that may have stuck out to them about that session in particular. Even if it isn't for the sake of improvement, any kind of conversation makes the subject feel more welcome, more trusting, and more comfortable with you as a hypnotist. Taking care of the subject and making sure they can be comfortable after the session is over is just as important as them being comfortable before and during the trance. If your subject is someone you may not know incredibly well outside of hypnosis, after your session may be a good time to try to get to know them better and become better acquaintances/friends. If not, there's no obligation to become friends with every person you have a session with. Even if you aren't set of maintaining a close bond with that subject, in particular, it's still probably a good idea to make sure they feel alright and take care of any questions or concerns they might have, if only out of obligation.

Of course, taking care of yourself after a session is important as well. Being able to notice what made you feel more confident, and what made you feel uncomfortable, will better arm you for your next session. If you said or did something that you know made your subject happy, but which didn't make you happy, talk more about it with them! Setting boundaries don't just apply to the subject in hypnosis—it also applies to the hypnotist's comfort zone and boundaries. Setting boundaries for yourself just as well as you set them for others sets you up for success in hypnosis when you don't work to only please others. Although it may not always seem like it, hypnosis is meant to benefit both parties, make them both feel satisfied, let them both have fun. If the hypnotist isn't enjoying a session because of something they're doing or have done to appease a subject, the session then loses some of its inherent value to the hypnotist.

The timeline of hypnosis, from before the trance to during the session to after waking up, is a set of times where the needs of both parties in the session need to be cared for psychologically. If either the hypnotist or the subject doesn't feel cared for, some might then consider that session a bit of a bust. Of course, taking care of the subject during the trance takes most of the attention, since that's the time where most of the "action" happens. However, the time before and the time after the session is over are also important times when both the hypnotist and the subject within the party should be checked on. Sometimes, there can be physical or psychological effects that can potentially damage the subject. Other times, all is well on the surface, but with no one to turn to for emotional comfort and conversation. Some subjects and hypnotists don't look for any kind of companionship after the session is over—they look the other way and go about their lives, and never interact with one another ever again. That way of behaving after a session is over is in no way shameful, but not all people are like that. Often, a subject or a hypnotist has something they want to share, a concern, or just someone to break the silence after a potentially dramatic session. Setting boundaries for yourself and sharing anecdotes or questions with your partner can drastically improve the way you feel about the session and whether or not the two people see one another again in the context of recreational hypnosis. Whether the subject has just come out of trance for the first time, or the subject has gone into trance dozens, or hundreds of times or the hypnotist has a concern they want to share, being able to dissolve that tension and treating the other person as more than the equivalent of a business partner, goes a long way in the satisfaction of both people in that relationship. Even platonically, the social factor or hypnosis is not one to be ignored. Although the physical and psychological nature of hypnosis is the parts of the science that so often get the most praise and the most attention, some may argue that the lasting impression of a certain session, certain trance, or certain person, is solidified in the minutes after the session is over. It may be that we all want such an intimate part of our minds being bared to bring us closer together as people. No matter how close or how far apart the hypnotist and subject may be, taking care emotionally of each other is something to be valued, on either side of hypnosis.

Chapter Nine:
Setting Boundaries For Yourself And Others

Being able to set boundaries for yourself, either as a subject or a hypnotist, is such an important part of hypnosis as a culture, which so often becomes overlooked because many people take it for granted. We treat boundaries strangely, in that many people imagine boundaries as static, things that don't ever change and which remain a defining factor a person. However, anyone you ever meet will likely have boundaries which change from session to session, from subject to subject. The boundaries we set for ourselves and the boundaries other people set for themselves almost always change are almost always subject to change, and always something that needs to be asked about before every single session. No matter how well you know the person you're working with, asking them about their boundaries and limits not only lets them know that you care about their comfort, but it also gives you an idea of where to take the induction. If a subject tells you that they have a bit of a problem with really harsh wording when it comes to hypnosis—they don't know why for sure, they just know that it makes them uncomfortable to be spoken to too professionally by a hypnotist—you, as their hypnotist, now know much more specifically how to phrase parts of your script so as to cater more toward that specific person and their preferences as a subject. Because you asked about their preferences/boundaries, you avoided what would've made that subject uncomfortable, even though you had only the best intentions as their hypnotist. As we communicate better with one another, we also learn how to best navigate through situations based on the other person, what we think they're probably going to say. Assuming is a fine thing to do with a person you know well when the situation doesn't involve hypnosis— although recreational hypnosis is in no way exclusively romantic, it is something very intimate, simply because it allows the hypnotist almost free reign of the mind of their subject. Because hypnosis is so intimate, many people may feel violated if their subject goes ahead and conducts themselves how they see fit without first consulting their subject, and accidentally hits a nerve during the session. It's that intimacy that's so often paired with extreme trust, which may have been violated since the hypnotist took for, granted the boundaries of their subject. A hypnotist can have pure and only good intentions at heart for their partner, but striking a chord by violating that trust and accidentally overstepping a boundary they didn't know existed can be the cause of a strained relationship between a hypnotist and their partner. Even if the hypnotist does ask about their subject's boundaries, no being careful to adhere strictly to them can cause problems between them and their subject. It can be hard to keep that note always in your head, though, and mistakes are made. If a subject is unwilling to forgive a single mistake that a hypnotist made in good but forgetful faith, that pair may not be suited well to each other. Keeping in mind the boundaries of your subject, even as a beginning hypnotist, likely puts you ahead of some of your peers who are also starting out as novice hypnotists. Taking the time to try and care for and cater to your hypnotist—while, of course, still minding your own boundaries and limitations—automatically sets you apart from at least some of your "competition".

Caring your subject that you care for their comfort and well-being, even just as a hypnotist and not as an acquaintance/companion, can genuinely go a long way with your subject, depending on their personality and how they respond to different levels of affection. In the sense of feeling comfortable, a big way to help someone to feel comfortable is to make them feel comforted. It's so incredibly important to listen and make your subject feel listened to and cared for, as you often don't know how much stress that subject is under. It can be hard to be constantly on the ball and listening to everything the subject has to say to you, but simply making them feel seen and acknowledged can go particularly far in making sure they understand that you're more and willing to listen to and adhere to their boundaries, no matter what they may be.

Of course, knowing a subject's boundaries and adhering to them throughout the entirety of the session are two very different things. Even if you register that a subject has a specific sensation or aesthetic or sensation that they want to avoid at all costs, you still have to utilize that information and be able to substitute anything in your script that may have collided with that boundary with something more suitable to that specific person. This can be hard, especially if you're the kind of hypnotist who exclusively writes their scripts beforehand and isn't used to making any kind of change right before the session begins. However, the ability to quickly creatively substitute those details out, as well as going that extra mile to take care of your subject and make them know that you've listened to them and are going to follow up on your promise to do everything you can to make them comfortable, also puts you considerably ahead of others who are beginning as hypnotists. Not to mention, your subject will also highly appreciate that gesture of kindness and compassion. If your subject hasn't outwardly told you before a session what their limits or preferences are, it's acceptable to simply ask them. Even if it sounds too blunt, it's much better to embarrass yourself for a moment then to purposefully avoid the question and later find out that you made your subject upset without even intending to. If your subject has boundaries that they've thought of, they should tell you when prompted. If, however, your subject doesn't have any specific boundaries that come to mind, allow them to think about it for a minute. If they can't think of anything, it's fine to proceed how you would have normally with the induction. However, along the way, periodically check in with your subject in a trance to make sure they're still comfortable. When going about this, make sure your prompting isn't so blunt that it pulls the subject directly out of the trance. If they're deeply entranced, simply slip in a "Nod your head/tell me 'yes' if you're comfortable and relaxed right now..." whenever you notice a large chunk of time in the session has passed. When bringing the subject out of trance afterward, check in on them again to ask if they felt uncomfortable at any point during the session. The answer would ideally by "no", but if it doesn't, understand what exactly pushes the boundary for your subject helps you better understand them and make the experience for them better if there's the next session with them. If there is going to be a foreseeable next session with that person, in particular, ask them to try and think of any boundaries they might have. Next session, when you get together, ask them if they've thought of anything. Continuing that process of thinking about your boundaries and how they've changed, if at all, helps the two of you come together and understand each other significantly better. It also helps you understand yourself much better, just taking a small chunk of time often to reflect on how you've changed and grown and whether or not any of those changes have a correlation with something that's happened recently in your life to place stress on you.

While the boundaries of the subject are certainly important, it's also very important not to neglect the boundaries and preferences of yourself, the hypnotist. Your boundaries also influence how you write up your scripts, how you behave toward your subject, and how you think of your sessions. Having an open conversation with your subject about boundaries can be a good way to not only be open about their boundaries but to be open about yours as well. If a subject you're seeing has a preference or a boundary which directly collides with your own, don't sacrifice your comfort and mental health for the comfort of the subject—although many people like to think that the more important person in a hypnotist/subject pair is the subject, the one who receives the most focus and the most instruction, the two people are evenly matched in importance. As such, don't let the desires and preferences of the subject obscure what you personally prefer and feel is best for yourself and your well-being. If the subject, however, directly interferes with those boundaries of yours, it's likely in your best interest and the best interest of the subject that the two of you cease seeing each other. Even if the subject is in no way directly harmful to you and has your best interests at heart the way you have their best interests at heart, it's likely that the two of you interacting in the context of a session could result in very unsavory results. Obviously, the ideal is a situation in which both the subject and the hypnotist want essentially the same thing out of each other. Of course, that happening is fairly uncommon, but it's something to be compromised on. Whether or not you're a hypnotist with very specific preferences and boundaries, or just someone who has a vague understanding of their partner's boundaries, compromising between yourself and your subject is one of the most important aspects of hypnosis.

Because we so often take communication for granted or fear that communicating properly will take away from the atmosphere of the session, many subjects and hypnotists simply don't communicate their concerns or their issues within the session to one another. Even when in trance, many subjects don't let their hypnotists know if they have a problem or feel uncomfortable. It can be hard to try and better communications when your subject simply doesn't seem to be able to bring themselves to communicating clearly—you can never force someone to speak clearly how they feel and why, but you can offer them a stress-free and calm environment where they can share their feelings, or at least be more likely to do so. Because people in the recreational hypnosis scene so often feel as though communicating an issue to their partner takes away from the ideal image of hypnosis, in which everything falls into place perfectly, they often don't feel comfortable expressing concerns about a session to their hypnotist, especially when in the middle of trance. Even the subconscious has a way of burying things that it doesn't want to be open about—this is where repressed memories come from. Because a lot of subjects feel much pressured to let everything fall into place on its own, many problems occur because of that miscommunication. When miscommunication happens, the relationship between the subject and their hypnotist can easily become more and more strained. When two people don't talk to each other even though they both know something isn't right, both parties get the feeling that they're being ignored. So, when in a position during a session where you feel uncomfortable for any reason, let the other person know as soon as you see fit. Whether it be right at that moment, or waiting until after the session is over, alerting your partner that something they've done affected you negatively is the only way they'll better understand you, your boundaries, and how to best take care of you as a subject/hypnotist.

There are some kinds of subjects, and some kinds of hypnotists, who naturally feel less compelled to open up to others about how they feel and why they feel that way, especially in the concept of something intimate, like hypnosis. This can be due to anything or nothing at all. Sometimes a subject will have issues at their home, with their friends or family, or some other kind of stress which puts them in an emotional position to close off. Other subjects are almost always closed off this way, possibly because of the way they were raised and possible because that's simply their personality. Even though it can be frustrating at time to have a subject who habitually doesn't open up to you, even if they have a problem, you can't get anywhere with that problem by pestering them to open up to you. It simply won't work, the more you ask and beg the subject to open up to you, the more they'll be turned off even from the idea of telling you when they have a problem that crops up, either inside a session or outside in their everyday life. While constantly pushing your subject to open up to you is usually not a very good idea, there are many ways that you, as a partner, can try and encourage them to be more open, like taking care of them whenever possible. This can work for many subjects, as they likely will instinctively want to return the treatment that you've been giving them. Even if you feel as if you're coddling them, placing them in a comforting and welcoming environment is exactly what someone who feels uncomfortable opening up needs—unless the subject openly recognizes what you're doing and asks you directly to stop. While comforting a person often does allow them to feel more willing to be open, some people just need more space and time than others to be able to open up to those around them emotionally. Additionally, when we treat a person a certain way for an extended period of time, the other person naturally begins to reciprocate. So after a certain amount of time spent going out of your way to care for your subject/hypnotist, that partner will soon find themselves caring for you as well, which leads to more communication. More directly, a partner is much more likely to communicate if you communicate with that incredibly often. Not so much that you may come off as obnoxious, but enough so that the partner gets the picture —communication is a massive part of how your relationships function, and you won't be sacrificing that anytime soon.

Often, we find ourselves in a place where we feel uncomfortable with something, but we aren't sure if it's a "valid" boundary to have or not. There are many things that people consider their boundaries, and which are subject to change because we grow out of those fears or sources of discomfort. Some people stick with the same boundaries their entire life. All subjects and hypnotists are different and will have different ways they face their limits/ boundaries. Some subjects aren't willing to acknowledge why they have what limits they do, and don't want to be pushed to think about them, although more subjects are able to consider the reasons they may have the limits that they do. All of those reactions are normal, and it's important to understand that even if you feel as though there's something off about your limits, or you actively want to change them, there are healthy and unhealthy ways to go about doing so.

Some ways that are unhealthy include:

a. Hiding your boundary from your partner because you think that it's subject to change – not only are your boundaries often a bit unpredictable, but there's no difference in importance between a boundary that you think is permanent and one that you think is temporary or subject to change. A temporary boundary is still on which correlates to how certain sensations make you feel—they're still a part of your comfort zone, even if that comfort zone is temporary. If you don't let your partner know what is and isn't good for you emotionally, even if only for one session, they know better how to move away from certain topics if they know that some specific content may cross one of your boundaries. It's never a good idea to hide any of your boundaries or limits from your partner within the session—ignoring your limit will only allow the cause for the boundary to grow stronger and control your life more. No matter you're the reason, it's always in your best interest as either a subject or a hypnotist, to tell the other person in the party about all the boundaries you have that could pertain to, or crop up during that session. If you avoid talking about them, you're only delaying whenever a problem will show up for you.

b. Just "sticking it out" and "manning up" – whether you're a man or not, being able to take the emotional high road for yourself and tell your partner is anything crosses a line or makes you uncomfortable is what will encourage them to do the same if the need ever arose. Showing your subject/hypnotist that you're more than willing to open up to them gives them a great example to follow, one that will help them also take care of themselves better in the long run. The concept of simply sticking it out if something makes you uncomfortable during a session, just dealing with it, stretches what you are and aren't willing to deal with that crosses your boundary. Stretching that boundary too far can have fairly harmful results for both you and your partner. So, not only is it important to tell your partner immediately if and when something crosses a boundary of yours, but it's also very important that when you set boundaries for yourself, set them hard. Having soft boundaries, ones that don't apply in certain circumstances or can be pushed around a little if need be allowed for not only a potentially malicious partner to take advantage of that, but it allows for your own comfort to be easily compromised by even a well-intentioned partner. Because you haven't drawn a clear line in the sand just yet as to how you know you want to be treated, the subject or hypnotist can only pick and choose and guess what might work for you. Setting harder boundaries allow for much more clarity when you work with someone else. This allows for much less miscommunication and much fewer understandings between the subject and their hypnotist. If they ask about boundaries, tell them your hard boundaries and say them firmly. Building up your sense of confidence in where you stand boundary-wise makes you more able to stand by those boundaries when the time comes. In the place of a hypnotist, being able to firmly say where your boundaries lie also makes you seem much more confident and surer of yourself, a green light for almost all subjects that you know what you're doing.

Some much healthier things to do include:

a. Being able to communicate clearly and frequently, maybe even a bit too much – communication is by far, the most important part of having a good relationship with your subject or hypnotist within hypnosis. Sometimes, you have to choose between shutting up and not saying anything about a concern or question you might have, and obnoxiously bringing up the same concern frequently in a string of conversation. Even if that conversation is one-sided, choose to be a bit obnoxious—communicating with your partner too much means a lot more than not communicating with them enough. Being able to annoy them a little is only an added perk to the pros of letting your partner know exactly what's up and why you want something changed, and anything else you may have a concern with. If that particular partner doesn't want to hear it out of you, tries to shut you down, or otherwise makes you feel guilty for trying to rise up a concern, it might be time to leave them as a hypnotic partner. It's possible that the way you're trying to communicate with that partner is unsavory, in which case it's important to take a step back and evaluate yourself, but if your partner doesn't want to deal with someone whose only intention is to communicate, that's on them and you'd be much better off with a partner who is much keener on active communication with one another. While very few people really appreciate a partner who's constantly in their faces disrupting the flow of conversation with information about themselves when the situation doesn't call for it, it's much better to have that situation than one in which a subjects emotional safety is put at risk because they decided to keep their boundaries locked up and didn't decide to let their hypnotist know about their limits. Not only is it simply a good idea, and not only do you have a responsibility and obligation to yourself to let your partner know when someone comes up, but you also have a responsibility to your partner to tell them about your limits, what you do and don't like. Telling them as soon as possible and reminding them could be the difference between a feel-good session and one that ends in a panic attack.

b. Taking time to reflect on your limits, and understanding them better – you don't have to keep all your trancing boundaries written down and locked up in a diary. Additionally, the reflection you have on yourself doesn't have to be everyday or every other day. It shouldn't be too often, actually, lest you get bored of it quickly however, it's always a good idea to take a moment and step back, looking at your boundaries objectively. While it obviously helps to better understand what exactly your boundaries are before you enter a new session with a potentially new subject or hypnotist, introspection can also help you better understand why you have those boundaries, where they come from, how they've changed over time, and how you can predict they'll change going forward. Having this kind of time where you can better understand yourself also allows you to more eloquently talk about boundaries with your partner. Encourage them to also take that time to sit back and think about themselves and their limits in the context of hypnosis. While not everyone can see immediate results or reach a new place of enlightenment after doing so, it still helps to clear the mind and to focus on what's important in the context of the session and your relationship with your subject or hypnotist.

Being able to focus on the best possible way to communicate with your partner opens up many ways to perfect the experiences that the two of you have with one another. Although the importance of communication and boundary is so often pushed aside, hypnosis may be considered a crime if there weren't such an emphasis on the importance of drawing a line in the sand. Taking the time you may need to consider your communication with your subject, their communication with you, and understanding how the two of you can improve and make the experience better mutually, shows that you are both responsible enough to call yourselves experiences hypnotists and subjects. Two people who can work together and make an experience better every time they repeat it—that responsibility is a trademark of both an experienced hypnotist, and a very good one.

Chapter Ten:
A Small Interlude About What It Means To Control Someone

There's most definitely something to be said about the actual appeal of hypnosis to many people—they get high off the idea of controlling someone else, even someone they may know and love. Their families, friends, or even complete strangers; there are many people who would relish in the idea of being able to control that person or those people. However, to approach hypnosis only with the goal of being able to control others minds, will only lead to disappointment.

It's more than likely that a random person's understanding of hypnosis is a bit more malicious than the idea of hypnosis to someone who actually has a background, or experience, in the field. Because hypnosis has become something of a horror trope—since you and I and everyone else on Earth are, on some level, afraid of being controlled against our will—many people avoid the idea of pursuing it all together. It can be scary, after all, to dive deep into the idea of letting someone else metaphorically poke around inside your mind. Baring your subconscious to someone requires a lot of trusts, and it's easy—and sometimes even tempting, in an intrusively thoughtful kind of way—to disregard the meaning of that trust and take advantage of the subject. Because of that risk that's always run whenever a subject goes into trance, many people steer far clear of the idea of hypnosis, let alone actually trying it out for themselves. Surely, it can be really terrifying to bare your subconscious, and your soul, to someone you may not actually know what well. If you ask anyone in your life who you know has trust issues, they may say that the idea of being hypnotized terrifies them. Luckily for them, most people with issues trusting people around them are not very easily taken into a trance. The most likely candidates for trance are people who very often wander off in their mind, and who are more open and trusting of others. So, if you're someone who experiences a lot of trust problems, or even paranoia, you're probably not at all in danger of being hypnotized anytime soon.

On another note, the morality of hypnosis is often called into questions by skeptics and those individuals who do suffer from a lot of trust issues—they wonder if a hypnotist should even be given the power over another person. After all, can't hypnosis quickly turn into mind control with the wrong person? Well, yes and no.

On the side of "no", no subject can be forced to do something they don't want to do or would never otherwise do. Asking someone in trance to strip down to their underwear in front of a crowd is not only amoral, but it probably wouldn't work, unless your subject was someone who was, for whatever reason, unfazed by that idea coming to life.

On the "yes" side, however, the point of hypnosis is to lower stress levels and help the subject mentally. This can often mean that the subject loses a lot of the inhibitions that may have had before being brought down into a state of trance. One in that mental state where all of their inhibitions are essentially gone, the doors are much more open for the subject to do many things they may not have otherwise done. The middle ground between the two is made up of things that the subject would never otherwise do for moral reasons, not for anxious reasons. The morals of a subject are never cast aside in trance, but things they worry about often are. A subject in trance could probably be "made" to send a text they never otherwise would. However, the subject wouldn't have otherwise sent the text because the idea made them anxious, not for any reason pertaining to their morals or conscience. So, while a subject can technically be made to do something they otherwise wouldn't do, they won't follow suggestions that tell them to perform actions that go against their basic moral code as a person. To be clearer, think of it this way —a person in trance can be made to do anything they might not otherwise do, but only when that suggestion is something they would do if they were incredibly intoxicated.

So, in a broad sense, being able to hypnotize people gives you some sort of power over others, if you choose to use that maliciously—of course, that power is limited to whatever the subject could find it in themselves to do, but it's not something which can be taken lightly nonetheless. Control is a funny thing when broken down to the reasons people seek it out. People who seek out the ability to control others often feel as though they're out of touch, or out of control, of themselves. They may have issues with someone in their inner circle, or trauma which causes them to lash out and seek a position in which they have control over the outcome of someone else's actions—to make up for the utter lack of control over their own. People who feel this way then, in turn, like to forcibly control others to obtain a power high they never would have otherwise experienced. Unfortunately for them, it's very unlikely that they'll really find the power they're so desperately searching out. There's really no basis to the idea we have about hypnosis being equivalent to "mind control". Although it's an intimidating idea on paper, there's no such thing that exists in the real world. There are certain subjects who are exceedingly suggestible, and there are subjects who have little boundary as to what they're not willing to do while in trance, but the only case in which you can "control" someone else's mind, is in which they previously give consent to have their mind "controlled", which, in a way, cancels out the very idea of having total control over a person's consciousness. It can be hard, most definitely, to achieve that kind of power high you may be looking for. However, it's unlikely that you'll find it through hypnosis. Hypnosis is structured in a way so that it can't be done in any capacity unless the recipient has consented in some way, shape, or form before the session has begun. That way, there's really no way for the recipient to be taken advantage of unless they consented to that exact treatment. Because trance can only be so strong, when a boundary is crossed, the trance will usually then immediately break and the subject will then return to fully alert state. So, unless the situation is part of a fantasy of that session, there's really no way to completely take advantage of a subject. This also applies to hypnotists who have no real intention to do their subjects any harm, they simply cross a boundary or get close to it—often the subject will immediately come out of the trance when they feel uncomfortable or in danger. Other times, the subject will stay in trance but in a lighter state of it. They may raise a concern but stay in a sort of trance. Even if they don't wake completely up out of the trance, any kind of concern raised by the subject means that, as a responsible hypnotist, you can no longer continue with that session. In a way, it's become void now that the subject has expressed their lack of satisfaction with something that has happened. After waking them up completely, make sure you both have each other's boundaries excessively clear, so as not to make that same mistake again.

It can be easy to make mistakes like that, and they luckily don't often result in adverse reactions that can be potentially dangerous to both the subject and the hypnotist. However, avoiding those mistakes and remembering to communicate shows your subject that you're committed to doing right by them and being a hypnotist who makes them feel safe and comfortable.

The illusion to many exists that hypnosis is morally grey, a way for a hypnotist who gains access and therefore, control, over their subject. Of course, this is untrue, but the fact that such a perception exists says something about the way that terrible people can try to manipulate their skills in hypnosis. Keeping yourself and your subject safe and comfortable, while remembering to communicate and adhere to each other's boundaries, should always be the top priority in that kind of relationship.

Chapter Eleven:
So You Think You Can Trance

As we progress through our lives, we gain the ability to better understand ourselves and our needs, both physical and emotional. Many of us have a desire to relieve ourselves from stress, in any way we can find. We seek out any kind of therapy we can get our hands on, try home remedies, and generally try to find any way we can to get better and feel better as soon as we physically can.

Suddenly, a new way to feel better arises—hypnosis, in which people open themselves up on the more intimate and barest level psychologically for the sake of relieving their stress. To the credit of hypnosis, such a thing does work for many people. There are a large number of factors that play into entering the hypnosis scene and flourishing.

For one thing, communication is the key. If you can't communicate properly with your subject or with your hypnotist, you might as well stop trying to advance in your hobby until you can better learn how to tell your partner what may be bothering you. That communication can pertain to setting boundaries for yourself or your partner, or it can revolve simply around a subject letting their hypnotist know that because of their risk for an adverse reaction, they ask that the hypnotist avoid certain phrases or imagery. No matter what, being able to calmly talk to your subject about some of the technicalities and conditions of your trance makes the entire experience much more enjoyable for people involved, hypnotist and subject. Additionally, knowing your subject fairly well increases the chance that the two of you will enjoy yourselves more than a pair who knows nothing about each other and has never met.

Something else massively important to take into consideration when trying to become a skilled hypnotist— being creative can make a world of difference to both your peers and your subject. Being able to plainly make up things on the fly, improve parts of inductions if need be, and use colorful and unique imagery to lull your subject into a trance, makes you a much more formidable competitor in the competition you might find yourself in with other people like you trying to become better at hypnosis. That creativity may take more time for some than others to harness and grow, but there's no shame in having to take some time to grow your skills manually. Creatively writing your own script doesn't come easily for most people, so consider it a gift if you do find yourself easily able to come up with things on the fly without any practice at it. Knowing your strengths and weaknesses can help you to massively grow your skills, compared to someone who improves upon all areas of their skill at once. Taking a moment to look at the way you do things objectively during your sessions, practicing on friends and family, and asking feedback and advice from both subjects you've worked with in the past and ones you have never worked with, greatly improves your chances of becoming an incredibly skilled hypnotist.

Of course, there are also some things to be wary of when becoming a hypnotist—there are many hypnotists who try to abuse their power, sometimes without even knowing that what they want to do qualifies as that abuse. While most all hypnotists have nothing but the best intentions at heart, it can be hard to discern those ignorant hypnotists from more malicious ones who seek out people they deem as weaker and easier to control.

No matter what cartoons you watched as a child may have told you, there is no such thing as genuine mind control. Even if you have a subject in a very deep trance, and the subject is incredibly suggestible, you still aren't technically directly controlling that person or their actions. While you're playing a very influential part in the actions, thoughts, and choices of that subject, a hypnotist is never truly in full control of their subject. Quite the opposite, in many cases—some people think of hypnosis as little more than a way for a hypnotist to allow a subject to be more open about what they want and why they want it. Many think of hypnosis as something more spiritual or psychedelic—something that helps a person open themselves up to a lot of their inner turmoil, which might help them face themselves more internally. Other people disregard this kind of thinking and take it as a merely clinical aid, something to help people who suffer from a lot of stress, anxiety, memory problems, and many other ailments. Hypnosis can be a source of healing for just about anyone who actively seeks it out. Although now hypnosis is looked upon by many with a bit of a skeptical eye, the process and the methods work just as well now as they did when hypnosis was medical magic in its own right. If anything, hypnosis is a much more profound way of aiding people than it ever was, if only because we now have a much better understanding of how it works.

In a way, hypnosis can be anything you make of it. If you want it to be something that allows you to control another person, so be it—although, you may not find much satisfaction in your findings as you try to verify what you find. If you want hypnosis to be something much softer and more wholesome, a kind of "home remedy" that anyone can learn, then so be it. However, be careful with how you think about hypnosis. Everything you think and perceive is always growing, changing, and evolving, so imagining your current perception as factual and/or static is foolish. Your mind will change, as will everyone's. The important thing about hypnosis is that the way your mind change is, in many ways, entirely up to you.

CPSIA information can be obtained
at www.ICGtesting.com
Printed in the USA
LVHW052102141220
674148LV00017B/3229

9 781513 668420